Natural Breast Enlargement

Through Effective Relaxation Techniques

Natural Breast Enlargement

Through Effective Relaxation Techniques

by
Joan Packard

FOREWORD
by William S. Kroger, M.D.

Cover Design by Michael Bolger

Jalmar Press
6501 Elvas Avenue
Sacramento, California

Printed in the United States of America

Library of Congress Catalog Number 80-83120

ISBN: 0-915190-30-3

Contents

Foreword

Joan Packard has written a stimulating and thought-provoking monograph on breast augmentation, a subject of great concern to many women in our society. Because we live in a culture oriented around the size, shape, and configuration of the breast, thousands of women attempt to achieve breast augmentation by physical, medical, and surgical measures.

As the author states, an increase in breast size can be achieved by a safe, inexpensive, and uncomplicated alternative to surgery. Furthermore, the method, according to her data and those findings presented by other pioneers in this field, has been demonstrated to be effective.

Natural Breast Enlargement, based on the author's master's thesis and on her success in private practice, makes use of hypnotic age regression, future time visualization, and suggestions to recall those sensations associated with developmental changes that occurred during puberty. These dynamics are well-established hypnotic phenomena and are based on the fundamental principles of classical conditioning and imagery conditioning. Images are the raw grist that feed the mills of reality. The brain stores all information in five senses. Because such data is retrievable, hypnosis allows subjects to tap forgotten assets and hidden potentials to transcend normal volitional capacities. These basic principles play an important role in the author's strategy for achieving satisfying breast augmentation.

The autonomic nervous system is not as involuntary as we have been taught in the past. Huge portions of its functioning can be controlled. Yet to ignore the obvious often is easier than to renounce the traditional. For instance, it is well recognized that "phantom" or spurious pregnancy (pseudocyesis) occurs in many women who have a strong desire for motherhood. Here we see all the concomitant signs or symptoms of pregnancy — endocrine hormones are released, the breasts enlarge, colostrum and milk appear in the breast tissues — all on the basis of the woman's imaginative capacities or fantasies stimulating the higher brain centers and the neuroendocrine apparatus.

Thus, every psychophysiological function is under control of cortical and subcortical centers (gray matter), that can effect, to some degree, alterations in end organ responses. The key to this process is relaxation, concentration, and imagery resulting in increased susceptibility to suggestions. Through practice, one can develop control over the type of autosuggestions that one concentrates on and imagines.

All individuals can be hypnotized to some extent, and everyone possesses the power of self-hypnosis or meditation. Highly motivated persons can harness, with practice, the power of imagery to do their bidding. I have used the principles of hypnosis and imagery conditioning for almost fifty years to reverse a large variety of psychosomatic disorders. *If these disorders can be produced, in part, by negative, harmful, or inappropriate thought processes, they can be reversed by substituting positive, healthy, and appropriate thought processes.*

In her master's thesis, Packard demonstrated through carefully controlled research that at the end of twelve weeks 71% of the women subjects were satisfied with their results; 64% perceived a difference in the size and shape of their breasts; 36% reported no perceived change; and 29% were dissatisfied with their results. Of the 36 subjects who agreed to participate, 31 finished the experiment including the post-treatment data; five subjects dropped out for one reason or another. The data were carefully evaluated by observations and questionnaires. Although results of this scientific research and documentation are not discussed in the book, the techniques described are based on the author's serious analysis of a very controversial and timely subject.

Natural Breast Enlargement is an essential alternative to surgery, and a *sine qua non* for anyone interested in breast augmentation by hypnosis and imagery conditioning.

William S. Kroger, M.D.
Author of *Hypnosis and Behavior Modification* and *Clinical and Experimental Hypnosis*

Preface

Natural Breast Enlargement is a book about the powers we all have within us to be what we wish to be. The techniques presented here can be applied to many other areas in your life — not just your goal of enlarging your breasts. I continually use these methods in my private practice where I counsel groups and individuals seeking personal growth, and self-improvement or assistance with situational and emotional problems.

Natural Breast Enlargement was not written to capitalize on the excessive concern about their breasts that pervades the lives of most women, or indeed on the chronic anxiety most of us live with concerning other aspects of our attractiveness. The basic reality about our breasts is that they are for feeding children. "Attractive" breasts are a myth created by society and sustained to a large extent by the media. I am not advocating perpetuating the "Playboy" stereotype of the ideal breast.

I believe that our bodies are OK regardless of size or shape; having large breasts, small waists, flat stomachs, etc. is not important. However, most women growing up in our society have a great deal of self-consciousness about their breasts that leads many of them to develop strategies to camouflage or reshape their breasts.

In 1978, according to the National Health Foundation, 25,000 women paid between one and four thousand dollars to have their breasts surgically enlarged through the insertion of silicon implants. Some estimates raise this number to almost 100,000 women. A high incidence of physical, cosmetic, and emotional complications also has been documented. The millions of dollars spent yearly on such surgical procedures, creams, breast exercisers and lotions state loudly and clearly that, for many women, having large breasts *is* important.

For these reasons, I feel that *Natural Breast Enlargement* is a much needed resource. Successful completion of the program will not necessarily improve your personality, whiten your teeth, or make your in-laws love you. Nevertheless, if you want a fuller bustline, no matter what your size or your motivation, you deserve a safe, uncomplicated alternative to surgery that is inexpensive, proven, and effective. You deserve to be what you want to be and I have written this book for you.

Dedicated to the thirty-one women who participated in my study. Working with you enriched my experience of "beautiful women."

Introduction

Ever since my tenth grade chemistry class I have been passionately interested in understanding how the mind works, what it can and cannot do. My interest began casually out of a discussion with several classmates over the meaning of the phrase "mind over matter." We speculated that if we only knew how to alter our molecular structures we could probably walk through the laboratory wall. The notion struck a responsive chord in me and I began to read everything I could find concerning the powers and limitations of the human mind. I delved into many subjects, including ESP, biofeedback, psychic phenomena, yoga, psychic healings, information processing, psychology, split brain research, and hypnosis. Although fascinated by what I read, I was also skeptical of the claims made in some of the non-scientific material about the power of the mind.

Then, in 1972, a severe weight problem led me to test out my skepticism. Months after the birth of my fifth child I weighed 195 pounds and was still wearing my maternity clothes! In desperation I decided to try hypnosis in order to lose weight. I had already tried every other known method of weight loss except having my mouth wired shut or submitting to surgical bypass. Hypnosis became my "last ditch" effort. When I was told by the hypnotist that I did not have to go on a prescribed diet, it was music to my ears. My skepticism, however, remained. How could I possibly lose weight without counting calories, weighing portions, and denying myself my favorite foods? I even went so far as to walk out of the session and head straight for the nearest fast food outlet for fried chicken, corn, rolls and honey! Nobody was controlling *my* mind and telling me what to do — not even ME!

Despite my initial rebellion, in seven sessions (three months' time) I lost thirty pounds and learned that, through relaxation and suggestion, I could lose weight — without dieting at all! I stayed at 165 for another six months, during which time my personal life underwent radical changes. Amazingly, I did not regain any of the lost weight. I then returned for two follow-up sessions, and, without consciously trying, lost an additional thirty pounds the following summer.

I was impressed.

I was so impressed that I began training in the use of hypnosis (under medical supervision) with the American Institute of Hypnosis in Los Angeles, and later with the American Society of Clinical Hypnosis. I reentered the academic world after an absence of fifteen years, and, in 1975, completed my bachelor's degree in psychology.

While in college, I volunteered at the Utah State Prison women's facility, teaching human sexuality and yoga. Following each class, I spent some time getting to know the women residents. On one such occasion, I spoke to a young woman who had just had her breasts surgically enlarged. I was surprised that a prison inmate would have the opportunity and resources to afford such a procedure.

The woman seemed eager to talk about her experience. She told me that she had volunteered to be a subject in an experimental operation involving a new type of breast implant. Although she claimed to like her larger breasts, she obviously was experiencing great discomfort and pain. The woman explained that she might have to return to the hospital for further surgery, although she wasn't sure why. This incident discomforted me and remained on my mind for sometime.

Two years later, while working on my Master's degree at California State University, *Ms Magazine* included in its September 1977 issue a special section on women and body image. I read about the 60% complication rate for surgical breast augmentation and the sizeable cost involved in the procedure. The "complications" ranged from infections, deformities, and excessive hardness, to painful and disfiguring scars and emotional difficulties. (In fact, a significant number of physicians currently oppose breast implant surgery on the basis of such unacceptably high complication rates.) Costs of the procedure ranged from

$1500 to $3500, literally adding insult to injury, as far as I was concerned. Remembering my own positive experience with weight loss, I felt angry that other women had to go through such an ordeal to achieve a sense of comfort and satisfaction with their bodies.

When I began to work on my Master's thesis, I found a culmination of my interest in the power of the mind and my belief in the value of self-improvement. While researching the topic of incest in *The Journal for Sex Research,* I discovered a study by James Williams demonstrating hypnosis as a successful method for stimulating breast growth.

All the pieces fell into place and I knew that I wanted to replicate the research to see if it really worked. I had been studying and practicing hypnosis for three years by then, and I felt confident that I could perform the task.

I soon learned that several other researchers also had investigated Williams' technique, and confirmed his results. Through my professional contacts in the field of marriage and family counseling, I knew of others who were developing similar programs.

Such breast treatments and studies, however, shared two features: every researcher was male and repeated statements were made that an increase in breast dimension correlated with an improvement in a woman's self-concept and sexual functioning. There was, however, no evidence to prove that these reported increases were caused by having larger breasts. In fact, at that time, I knew of no studies that demonstrated a relationship between poor sexual participation and enjoyment with breast size. I was curious to see if such claims were accurate (I felt they were misleading) or if they were a consequence of male bias. Would a female researcher have similar results? I decided to replicate the breast enlargement studies to investigate such questions. With my chairman's approval, I proceeded to develop a replication of Williams' 1974 study.

Natural Breast Enlargement is an outgrowth of that work.

Chapter 1

THE INHERENT GIFT

If you're a woman who has longed for a fuller, firmer contour to your breasts or for larger breasts, I want you to know right now **you deserve larger breasts and you can have larger breasts.** Regardless of what you may have heard or read, the only "reason" that is important to having larger breasts is really wanting larger breasts.

You have within you the ability to enlarge your breasts safely and naturally. You can begin today to develop that inherent gift and augment the size of your breasts. The ability is not magical or mysterious or difficult. It is easy, safe, and lasting.

The method described in this book is not for everyone. Some women are so discouraged by *un*successful breast enlargement methods that they have given up hope. You, however, have already proven yourself — you have this book in your hand. You have shown the interest and desire to start on a fascinating adventure.

Before you are through with this chapter you will be on your way to learning a safe, easy, and practical method that will bring you the breast size you have dreamed of and results that are permanent.

How is this possible?

Read on, and I will demonstrate that you already possess the two ingredients essential to successful breast enlargement: the ability to relax and the ability to pretend. The Natural Breast Enlargement program consists of applying these talents daily over a period of time to achieve the results you desire.

Let's Relax

Join me now in a simple warm-up exercise. Read the following instructions. Review them if you need to. Then, put the book aside and begin.

Sit comfortably in your chair with your hands in your lap, close your eyes, take a deep breath and hold it. Now exhale, and as you exhale allow your body to relax. Repeat the process. Take another deep breath, hold it, and as you exhale count backwards from ten to zero and with each count tell yourself that you are relaxing more and more. Notice how good this feels. You may be aware that your heart is pumping more slowly or that your breathing is now effortless or it may have speeded up. Notice how relaxed you are. As you say the number zero let your body go completely limp. Enjoy this pleasant state for a few moments. When you are ready, take another deep breath, open your eyes and be aware of how rested you are.

What you have just done is basic to increasing the size or changing the shape of your breasts: it is the process of relaxing your body and quieting your mind.

Let's Pretend

Whether you want to enlarge your breasts a little bit or a lot, your mind plays a vital role in reaching your goals. How you use your mind is the important factor.

You have had the ability to pretend since your first moment of birth and you have used it all your life, although you may not have been aware of it.

You used your power when you:

- Prayed and had your prayers answered;
- Thought about purchasing a new car, checked out the models and prices, and then bought one;
- Told yourself that something terrible was going to happen to you and it did;
- Cried during a sad scene at the movies and felt badly.

These situations are simple examples of the incredible power of your subconscious mind. They illustrate a powerful and persistent concept that is the core of the breast enlargement program:

ANYTHING YOU HOLD IN YOUR MIND AND DWELL ON BECOMES REAL

Impossible? Not at all.

Your subconscious mind works in a wonderful way; it takes everything literally and is concerned only with end results. Your subconscious, like your nervous system, cannot tell the difference between what is real and what is imagined as "real." It simply reacts to information that you give it.

To demonstrate my point, I want you to use your imagination to do the following exercise:

Imagine yourself standing in the kitchen and holding a lemon that you have just taken from the refrigerator. The lemon feels cold in your hand. Examine the outside of it and notice its bright yellow skin. Squeeze it a bit and feel its waxy firmness and weight. Now raise the lemon to your nose and smell it. Nothing smells quite like a sour lemon, does it? Now cut the lemon in half and as you do the juice squirts out a bit and the aroma is stronger. Now bite deeply into the lemon and swirl the juice around in your mouth.

By this time, if you have allowed your imagination full power, you are probably aware of a great deal of saliva in your mouth as your body responds to the images you created in your mind.

Thoughts. Mere thoughts affected your salivary glands. The thoughts did not reflect reality but rather something that you imagined.

When you read the preceding paragraph about the lemon, your mind believed and accepted that you had a lemon even though you really did *not* have one. Your brain responded literally to the message and said to your salivary glands, "Hey, she's biting a lemon, hurry up, wash it away."

Simple and powerful isn't it? Through the natural power of your imagination and your suggestibility you created a physical response within your body. If I had said to you, "Make your mouth water, please," you would have had a difficult time making saliva flow, and you might even feel like you suddenly had a mouthful of cotton balls. The ability to imagine and pretend is the second ingredient in the method you will use to increase the size of your breasts.

The Natural Breast Enlargement program consists of the steady repetition of relaxing and pretending over a period of time until you reach your desired breast size and shape. Whatever you think about and pretend is true becomes a reality. You do not need conscious effort or willpower. You have nothing to lose by using your mind to increase the size and shape of your breasts.

The Mind Does It All

Enlarging your breasts is safe, easy and natural. It just happens. It happens as easily as reading this page or wondering what time it is or thinking about the opposite sex. Remember this about the method:

— It is not mysterious
— It is not supernatural
— It is not philosophical
— It is not positive thinking
— It is not occult
— It is not willpower

Quite the contrary:

— It is scientific
— It is natural
— It is comfortable
— It is effortless
— It is safe
— It works

Natural Breast Enlargement is scientifically and medically sound and has already been used successfully by a large number of women, aged 18 and over. You can do it, too.

I have included many exercises throughout the book in order to teach you the nuts and bolts of the process, and to allow you to experience the resources and powers you have within you. If you content yourself with "knowing" you could experience an exercise and choose not to perform it, you will finish the book with a possibility, not an actuality. If your curiosity leads you to try the program before it is fully presented, then you will be building the second floor before the first has been finished and your results may not be satisfying.

Ultimately there is no way to know if this process really works for you except to do it. Unless you have some experience of your own that validates what is written here, then you have little else to go on but my say-so, which may be totally meaningless to you.

These techniques are not to be used in place of adequate medical care. You are wise to have a routine and yearly breast examination by your doctor as well as special breast examinations when you are taking birth control pills. In case there are any doubts about your health in connection with your breasts, always consult your doctor first before starting on this program.

Practice Exercise #1

For now, though, do the following exercise and start to get results from Chapter one:

> Sit comfortably, close your eyes, and imagine yourself starting Chapter two. See yourself interested and absorbed and convinced that you have the power within you to alter the size and shape of your breast. See yourself lying down and doing each exercise called for.

Chapter 2

THE POWER OF SUGGESTION

You have just gotten out of the shower. As you dry your body you catch a glimpse of yourself in the bathroom mirror. You are vaguely aware of your body. Perhaps you admire what you see reflected there. More likely, as your eyes travel over your form, you merely glance at your breasts trying to avoid the reality that the mirror presents. There is nothing really upsetting, just a tiny brief message to your subconscious that your breasts don't count.

You dress and you have a hazy awareness of some discomfort as you notice that you don't quite fill your clothes the way that you would like. Maybe you also feel a bit annoyed that it should matter to you at all. No big deal, and so another negative message about your breasts is delivered to your subconscious.

During the day you will experience directly or indirectly a variety of messages from TV, magazines, billboards, and books all testifying to the desirability and importance of having large breasts. Just in case a new car couldn't be farther from your mind, a seductively clad, full-breasted woman in a magazine ad or TV commercial reminds you that beautiful cars and beautiful bodies go hand and hand.

The message that well-developed breasts are important is communicated in more subtle ways, too. Perhaps you will notice (and pretend you didn't) any woman with breasts larger than yours and feel just a twinge of envy that you don't look like she does. You can't miss the obvious glances of many men when they see a woman with large breasts. Nor can you miss their barely concealed remarks that appear to verge on worship of the female breast.

Here is suggestion in its most subtle form. The ideas are introduced indirectly, discretely and gradually and you have no conscious awareness that your concept of your breasts is being influenced. The messages find their target despite your unlistening ears or your disinterested eyes. They travel along your nerves to your subconscious memory storage where they wait patiently for an appropriate moment to intrude into your consciousness.

Your subconscious is a limitless storehouse of suggestions and impressions. Throughout your entire life, your mind has been taking a complete, stereo high fidelity full color movie of each instant, complete with vision, hearing, touch, smell, taste, and emotions. Every thought you have, every action you take, every impression you receive, causes some response in your brain structure and this change is permanently recorded. The subconscious forms an imperishable record of everything you have experienced, thought, or done in the past, and exercises an influence over you, building up your present knowledge and guiding your everyday actions.

Your subconscious is very efficient. It always responds at the right moment with the proper instruction from the appropriate storage bin of recorded information. What you call "common sense" is nothing but a reservoir of experiences out of which your judgments flow, while the experiences themselves are hidden away in the subconscious depths of your mind.

You Cannot Escape The Influence of Suggestion

You are constantly receiving suggestions about the acceptability of your breasts. From infancy on, you probably have received many negative suggestions about your breasts; and, not knowing how to thwart these suggestions, you unconsciously accepted them as true. The process has been going on in every woman's life since day one. The impact has been heightened (however unintentionally) by friends, family and your own increasing self-consciousness about your budding womanhood.

Remember the first time you heard the sexual snicker? Usually it was made by laughing and wise-cracking adolescent males speculating on the measurements of another girl.

"Ya think she's a 36?"

"Nah, 35, maybe, but definitely not a 36."

During treatment for breast enlargement, one physician found that such belittling remarks were interpreted as suggestions, and were definite factors inhibiting breast development during puberty. One woman, as a child, had wished that she was a boy because her parents had wanted a boy and had let her know that when she was very, very young. She never forgot it.

Most of the women in my breast development study (discussed in Chapter three) reported similar experiences. Only three women out of the thirty-one I treated said they had felt proud about their developing breasts. All the others indicated they had been ridiculed or made to feel ashamed.

Another woman in my study reported her brother whisked a copy of a "girlie" magazine out of her sight, and the embarrassed silence that followed made her wonder what was going on. She said, "I was curious, so a few days later I found the magazine and a funny feeling came over me as I looked at the naked bodies of those women. I was fourteen then and it seemed to me my breasts had stopped growing. I knew that I would never look that good. I have been comparing my body to those of other women ever since and I figure every man that looks at me is comparing me to those pictures." Zap! Another message to your subconscious — large breasts are where it's at! — and you don't have them!

Your subconscious will not argue with you or talk back to you. It doesn't say "That's not true" or "having larger breasts isn't important." The anxiety and emotional upset felt by that woman over the size of her breasts and the statements made to her about them became factors influencing and interfering with the natural physical processes necessary to develop her breasts to their optimum size.

Just as you are susceptible to being influenced by others' suggestions, you also are susceptible to being influenced by your own thoughts. There is no exaggeration in saying that all of you have been influenced by negative suggestion to some extent, either by ideas you have accepted uncritically from others or ideas you have convinced yourselves are true.

Let's talk now about effectively blocking those unwanted negative suggestions and reprogramming your mind with new suggestions or affirmations to achieve the results that you want. Whether you want to enlarge your breasts a little or a lot, your mind, through your suggestions to yourself, plays a vital role in reaching your goals. How you use this power is an important factor in increasing the size of your breasts.

If You Thought It, You Can Unthink It

Whatever you think and hold to be true in your conscious mind will, if held long enough, sink into your subconscious mind. Then your subconscious will use its enormous power to fulfill the image created by your thoughts.

You deserve larger, fuller, shaplier breasts and you can have them. It's as simple as that.

Thinking you're small will keep you small.

Thinking you're larger will make you larger.

If your thoughts always are dwelling on the fact that your breast size is inadequate, then you are dwelling on their inadequacy, whether you realize that or not. You have become head cheerleader, rooting for your inadequate breasts. Now start rooting for the other team. Imagine your breasts as larger, fuller, and firmer.

The poor get poorer because they hold poverty pictures in their minds. The rich get richer because they hold pictures of future profits in their minds. Imagine what would happen to a millionaire if she kept imagining the worst. Try thinking that you are small *and* large breasted, together, at the same time — you can't do it! You cannot hold these two thoughts simultaneously in your mind because the mind can focus only on one thing at a time. So choose, which will it be for you? **You are what you say you are.**

Through the simple processes described in the following chapters, you will learn how to reject the negative suggestions you unknowingly accepted and open the channels of your mind to enlarge your breasts. This process takes a few minutes each day, the know-how, and the willingness to use it. Success should come easily to those of you who have gone through the effort of trying various breast enlargement devices, only to suffer the pangs of frustration and dismay as they proved ineffective.

One young woman in my study said,

"My breasts began to develop when I was eleven. All my friends had already developed and I was embarrassed around them. I was always trying something to improve the appearance of my chest. First I used kleenex stuffed into my bras and finally when I was seventeen I sent away for a breast exerciser. I used it faithfully for two weeks, just like the exerciser book suggested and after that time I couldn't tell if any improvement had been made or not. I got discouraged and gave it up."

After three months, using the Natural Breast Enlargement suggestions found in Chapter nine, she had increased her breast measurements from 32¼ inches to 34½ inches. She was delighted the day she went out to buy a new larger bra.

Reprogramming your mind to increase the size of your breasts involves using your suggestibility by talking to your subconscious mind effectively in a passive, relaxed state. By talking to your subconscious mind you can direct your conscious mind so that it presents as little resistance as possible.

Your present thoughts about your breasts were formed without effort or any sense of strain. You can use the same process in forming new thoughts in an effortless condition. The suggestions around you, in and of themselves, have absolutely no power over you except the power you give them. To enlarge your breasts you have to give your mental consent. And that is true about the suggestions you are reading now. First you entertain the thought, then it becomes yours. You have the capacity to choose. If you want to enlarge your breasts choose to enlarge them in your thinking.

Practice Exercise #2

Sit comfortably in your chair. Quiet your mind and relax your body as you learned to do in Chapter one.

In your mind's eye, bathe your body in a beam of brilliant white light. Imagine yourself wearing a very special dress or blouse you have always wanted to wear with larger breasts. Imagine seeing your reflection in a mirror. Enjoy seeing yourself in the dress for a moment. See it happening — as if it were true. Allow yourself this moment of "make believe."

Seeing and Believing

You have just taken a very important step: you have used the power of your mind to set in motion the creative forces that will bring about exactly what you have pictured. The thought triggers the subconscious mind to get busy and work its "magic."

— You want it to happen.
— You expect it to happen.
— You feel it happening to you.

Right now, by seeing and believing the image of the new you, you began to bring about the changes you desire. Suggestion works on you whether you are aware of it or not. If you see it and hear it, the suggestion has been made and is being stored in your subconscious to become a part of your future. If you see it and don't hear it, or if you hear it and don't see it, the suggestion process will still take place — the suggestion will still reach your subconscious. Your own imagination implements the suggestions in order to effect the changes in yourself.

Most suggestions you give yourself will be pleasant ones. You enjoy picturing yourself in your attractive new clothes, seeing yourself gaining admiration among your friends and being more attractive to yourself.

All of these pleasant mental pictures, entertained while in an enjoyable state of deep relaxation, in effect reset the motivating mechanism within you from position A, that has made you what you are today, to position B, that now makes you what you want to be.

This kind of programming automatically works for your benefit — always and unceasingly.

Believe it.

Expect it.

Chapter 3

WHAT MAKES THE PROCESS WORK

One of the most fascinating features of your subconscious mind is that you usually are unaware of its acting. You do not consciously control the beating of your heart, your digestion, the elimination of your food, the circulation of your blood or the temperature of your skin. All of these and other vital bodily processes are controlled by your autonomic (involuntary) nervous system. Whether you are awake or asleep, your subconscious tirelessly regulates all the necessary functions of your body without any help from your conscious mind. As you read these words, your subconscious mind is causing your eyes to blink frequently enough to keep them moist. Your eyes are changing their focus continuously and the black and white marks on which you are focusing are being transformed to words, meanings, and ideas. Imagine the chaos that would result if you had to pay attention and consciously control each of the foregoing activities!

Only recently has scientific research begun to recognize the potential that the mind has for influencing bodily functions previously thought to be beyond conscious control.

Mind Power

Scientists traditionally have treated the disturbances of our normal bodily functions chemically. Some recent research, however, has demonstrated that the *mind alone* has the power to affect blood flow, heart-rate, pain, tissue growth, and even counteract the known effects of certain drugs.

In an experiment involving a group of medical students, for example, a powerful sedative was injected intravenously in amounts that should have made them very sleepy and listless. However, the students were first placed in a state of deep relaxation and told that the drug would have no effect. Shortly after the administration of the sedative, the group was tested on spatial, motor, and neuro-muscular relations. Everyone in the group remained awake and alert and performed in a perfectly normal manner. Several days later the same medical students were given very small amounts of the identical sedative without being put in a state of deep relaxation and were told nothing. Later, during the same testing, not one of them was able to perform the identical tests and several actually fell asleep trying.

Dr. Herbert Benson of Harvard University, author of *The Relaxation Response,* has demonstrated that simple relaxation procedures can produce changes in the autonomic nervous system, such as reduction of high blood pressure or the relief of anxiety. Other researchers have demonstrated the possibility of using the mind to improve vision, control allergies, remove warts, and influence directly or indirectly a wide variety of emotional, physical, and psychological functions.

If thought can produce such amazing results it is not surprising that thoughts can enlarge your breasts.

The process that produces the changes is the repeated use of imagery and suggestion while your mind and body are deeply relaxed. No physical effort is involved.

YOUR BODY REACTS TO YOUR THOUGHTS

Mind is where the action is
Body is where the reaction is

Your mind affects your body and your mind and body always work together to produce results. You have already had a simple demonstration to that effect when you imagined the lemon in Chapter one. The key is to turn the job over to your subconscious. Most people don't do that because they do not have enough trust in their automatic mental faculties.

At the Menninger Clinic, Elmer and Alyce Green conducted research with migraine sufferers. During a migraine headache, the blood vessels in the head dilate, and the blood vessels in the hand contract. No one knows why this happens, only that it does happen. The Greens found that when they taught migraine sufferers to raise their hand temperatures ten to twenty degrees with biofeedback techniques, the sufferers had fewer and less painful headaches. Some people had no success at all in raising their hand temperature — they were "skeptical of the training, or suspicious that hypnosis was being used, or very self-determined." People who TRIED, failed. In fact, the physical changes were exactly opposite from what they wanted — their hands got colder and their headaches worsened. They did not trust their own minds to produce the effect they wanted. Passive willingness and a neutral or non-resisting attitude by some sufferers were important factors in the successful reduction of their painful headaches.

The Breast Enlargement Studies

In 1974, James Williams reported in *The Journal of Sex Research* his successful completion of a simple nonsurgical technique for increasing breast size, using three functions of the mind:

Relaxation: the process of quieting your mind and releasing the tensions from the body.

Suggestibility: the power of suggestion to affect behavior and bodily functions.

Visual Imagery: the ability to create pictures in your mind.

Williams conducted a pilot study (like a test run) and a main study (the real thing). Measurements of each woman's breast, including vertical, horizontal, and circumferential measures, were taken under controlled circumstances. In the pilot study, three women were given weekly relaxation treatments but no suggestions for breast development. At the end of the twelve weeks, women who *had* been receiving suggestions for breast development increased their breast measurement an average of $1\frac{5}{8}$ inches, whereas the women exposed to relaxation alone showed no change.

Thirteen women who desired larger breasts took part in the main study. All the women received twelve weekly treatments consisting of relaxation and repeated suggestions to feel again the sensations in the breasts that occurred during puberty. They also were to picture themselves at some time in the future and visualize their body-image with increased breast size. When the research was completed the increase of the women who participated ranged from 1 inch to 3½ inches. The average increase for the group was 2.11 inches.

Two similar studies by Dr. Richard Willard of the Institute of Behavioral and Mind Sciences, and Allan Staib and D. R. Logan of the University of Houston reported in the *American Journal of Clinical Hypnosis* equal success with the breast enlargement technique. Staib and Logan also conducted a three-month follow-up on the women participating in their study and reported that an average of 81% of the gains in breast size had been retained.

An Effective and Inexpensive Method

I conducted similar research in 1978 and confirmed for myself that here was a safe, simple, and effective method to increase breast size. My study was composed of two basic elements. The first was a questionnaire given both before and after the 12-week treatment, investigating such areas as: body-image satisfaction, self-esteem, feelings about sex and the body, and about pre-adolescent and adolescent years. I also conducted an interview in conjunction with the pre-questionnaire to explore each subject's menstrual history, early family life, attitudes and reactions at the time of early breast development, and motivation for participation in the study. The information gained from these inquiries proved to be helpful and interesting and will be referred to at various times throughout the book.

The second element was the treatment itself. Thirty-one women volunteers ranging in age from 19 to 43 years were divided randomly into four different treatment groups and given a weekly relaxation treatment and suggestions for breast development for a period of 12 weeks. I modified the breast enlargement suggestions of the previously published studies in order to evaluate the effectiveness of the three types of suggestions the researchers had used.

The suggestions for each treatment group were as follows:

1) CONTROL: subjects received three suggestions: remembering the time when their breasts were first developing, followed by feeling various sensations in their breasts, and finally

picturing themselves at some future time and seeing their body-image with the breast size they desired.

2) AGE REGRESSION (AGEREG): subjects received repeated suggestions to remember the time when their breasts were first developing.

3) BREAST GROWTH (BRGR): subjects received repeated suggestions to feel various physical sensations in their breasts.

4) FUTURE TIME VISUALIZATION (FTV): subjects received suggestions to picture themselves at some time in the future after the study was completed and visualize their increased breast size.

Each subject's weight and breast measurements were taken weekly, including a chest measurement taken just under the breasts. The latter was a control measure to be sure the breast measurement was not due to an increase on the back or upper torso.

At the end of 12 weeks of treatment, Group 4 (FTV) had the largest amount of increase, ranging from .85 inches to 1.19 inches. Group 2 (AGEREG) followed with a range of .57 inches to .99 inches. Groups 1 (CONTROL) and 3 (BRGR) increased the least with a range of .25 inches to .64 inches. One woman in Group 3 had an increase in breast measurement of 2 inches. However, she was the only woman in those two groups to achieve such a significant increase.

The most interesting measurement was the one taken of the chest just under the breasts. *Every* woman had a *decrease* in this measurement ranging from 3/4 to 1¼ inches, regardless of how little or how much they increased their breast measurement. One woman lost eight pounds and I expected to see her breast measurement decrease significantly by the end of the treatment. *It didn't, it remained the same!*

Frequent Visualization is the Key

Increase in breast size was not related to age, marital status, number of children or being on birth control pills. Two women who had had hysterectomies prior to participation in the study increased their breast size 1 inch and 1¼ inches respectively.

The most powerful factor affecting breast growth was the frequency of visualization. This result is consistent with those of the previous studies. The more a person thinks about and vividly imagines the suggested effect, the less they believe that it *cannot* occur. More simply stated, **suggestions are effective only to the extent that they become self-suggestions and are not being contradicted.** Group 4 (FTV) reported imagining themselves with larger breasts 50% more often than all the other groups. Group 1 (CONTROL) said they visualized only "sometimes" and "rarely."

I genuinely was surprised at such a result because the subjects most highly motivated to increase their breast size (Groups 1 and 3) visualized the least and their increase was rather small. The women in Groups 4 (FTV) and 2 (AGEREG), whose motivation for participation primarily was an interest in using their mind to affect the body, visualized most frequently and their increase was quite significant. This information was particularly surprising since all the women were assigned randomly to groups and statements about motivation were gathered prior to the first treatment.

Belief in the method of breast enlargement did not appear to have an effect on whether their breasts enlarged or not. Although the women in Group 4 (FTV) achieved the largest increase in breast size, they only "slightly believed" that this method of relaxation and suggestion would enlarge their breasts. On the other hand, Group 2 (AGEREG) women, whose increases were similar to those of Group 4, stated that they "strongly believed" relaxation with suggestion would enlarge their breasts.

Let Go of Your Doubts

One final element that seemed to have influenced the degree of breast enlargement was doubt. During the course of treatment an interesting thing happened. Breast measurements from sessions 1 through 4 showed a steady increase in breast growth. However, measurements taken during session 5, 6, and 7 appeared to decrease slightly for all groups. Then during sessions 8 through 12, the measurements reflected a steady increase for Groups 4 (FTV) and 2 (AGEREG), but only a minimal increase for Groups 1 (CONTROL) and 3 (BRGR). I discovered in the "reactions to treatment" questionnaire, administered following completion of the research, that the women in Groups 1 and 3 did not feel they were growing *fast enough* and this belief was shared by all the subjects in those two groups. The women in Groups 4 and 2 did not reveal this element of doubt. Thus sustaining an elaborate pattern of imagining (larger breasts) while at the same time focusing on information that contradicted the image (not growing fast enough) served to defeat the purpose. Scientific research reports that when subjects do not experience a suggested effect, they tend to discontinue focusing on the suggestions and instead evaluate and criticize their performance. In so doing, they deny the reality or truth of the suggestions.

One of the primary purposes for administering the pre- and post-questionnaire was to determine if a relationship existed between breast increase and an increase in sexual participation and enjoyment, as many other researchers had reported. My results did not show any significant increase in satisfaction or interest in sex, frequency of sexual intercourse, or frequency of enjoyment of sex.

The strongest motivation for increasing the size of their breasts came from the women themselves. None of them desired breast enlargement to please someone else. According to their responses on the questionnaire, 87% of the women did not suffer from either low self-esteem or a poor body-image. Wanting to have larger breasts was a matter of personal preference.

If *your* personal preference is to have larger breasts, or just fuller, firmer, and shapelier breasts, decide now to use the Natural Breast Enlargement Program. The only "reason" that is important is your own desire to have your breasts be the way you have always wanted them to be. You're worth it. You deserve it.

Practice Exercise #3

Say the following affirmation to yourself; memorize it. Repeat it eight times while relaxing as you've already learned how to do. You are on your way to a lovelier you.

> I am excited by my goal of wanting larger breasts, and I win the support of others to achieve my goal. I am expressing my true self in my desire to have larger breasts.

Chapter 4

HOW YOUR BREASTS DEVELOPED

Understanding the physical structure of your breasts will help you realize why pills, creams, hormone preparations, nutritional supplements and exercisers all have a minimal effect, if any, on altering the size of your breasts.

Your breasts consist of milk ducts, glandular tissue, fatty tissue and connective tissue, all of which are generously interlaced with blood vessels and nerves and are held in a natural "bra" of skin. They are located on the front side of your chest with each breast extending from the first or second rib to the sixth or seventh rib.

Your breasts are not like your arms or legs. They are modified sweat glands called mammary glands, the primary function of which is to produce milk to feed children. Your breast is composed mostly of glandular tissue that receives nutrients and hormones through an extensive network of blood vessels. There is also a larger percentage of fatty tissue throughout the breast (even in small breasts), that determines its size and form. That is why when you lose weight the breasts are often the first place to show the loss. The fatty tissue seems to insulate and protect the complex system of milk ducts which open up on the nipple.

There is no major system of muscles or ligaments within your breasts to keep them in position. There are, however, small muscles in the areola and nipple which are responsible for the nipple's erection when stimulated.

Your breasts are separated from your chest muscles by connective tissue called *fascia.* Unfortunately, a misguided notion that there are muscles *within* the breasts and that developing them will lead to breast enlargement has led many women to employ breast developers without noticeable results. The development of the chest muscles merely gives the illusion that the breasts have enlarged.

Similarly, dietary supplements are geared to increase the fatty tissue in the breast. Unfortunately, there does not seem to

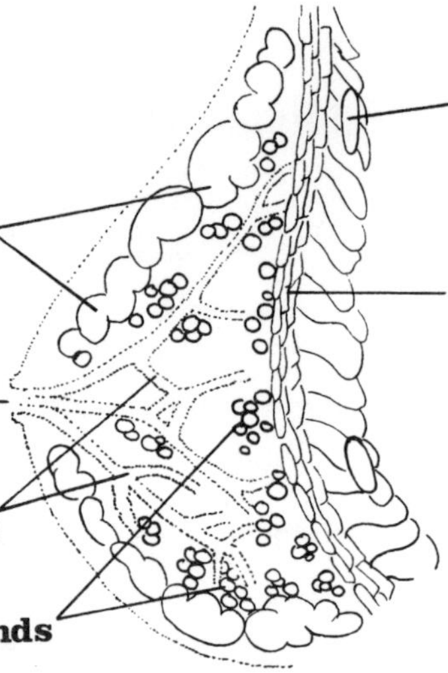

be a way to increase the breasts' fatty tissue without also increasing other fatty tissue throughout the body. So, you get larger breasts *and* a larger body. A fat body is a questionable price to pay for larger breasts.

The Influence of Hormones

Two major hormones are responsible for the development of the breasts. Estrogen and progesterone, when present in sufficient quantities and balance, cause your breasts to develop — usually at the onset of puberty. When an estrogen cream is rubbed into the breast there may be a stimulation in the nipples but there is little, if any, in breast growth. Your hormones also are responsible for changes in breast size during pregnancy, when nursing a baby, or when you are taking birth control pills.

Your breasts change at different stages of your life. In childhood, breast development is about equal for males and females. During puberty your breasts increase rapidly from a budding stage to a mature state. Most of the changes inside are caused by an accumulation of fat and the effect of the various hormones, not all of which are completely understood. The size, shape, and weight of your breasts fluctuate often, and are affected by menstruation, heredity, age, weight gains and losses, pregnancy, and, as with all other soft tissue in your body, the relentless pull of gravity.

The Influence of Emotions

Almost every woman develops breasts to some degree. But, for some, the breasts never get beyond the "bud" stage. They simply do not mature. One explanation for this, according to many authorities, is that early breast development is influenced markedly by emotional and psychological factors. Sometimes your conscious mind can interfere with the normal rhythm and functioning of these processes by worry, anxiety, fear or depression. Menninger Clinic researchers Elmer and Alyce Green and Dale Walters assume that "every change in the mental or emotional state, consciously or unconsciously, goes hand and hand with an appropriate change in the physical state; conversely, every change in the physical state goes hand and hand with an appropriate change in the mental and emotional state whether it is conscious or unconscious."

BUD STAGE **PUBERTY** **MATURITY**

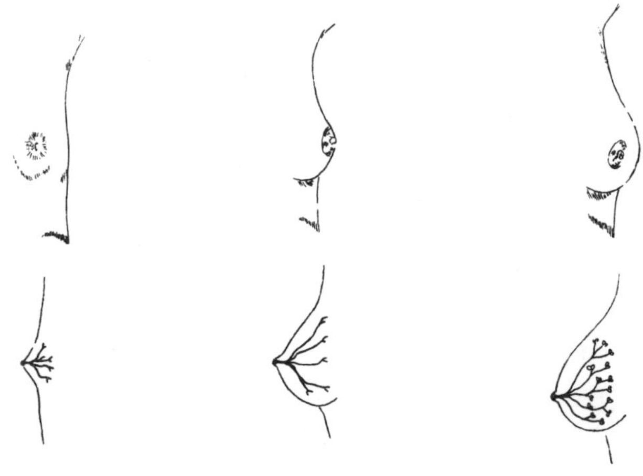

Severe emotional stress, such as fear, an unhappy home atmosphere, or the death of a loved one, is capable of throwing the hormones out of balance and delaying breast development, sometimes indefinitely. Thoughts come and go; emotions last for some time.

For example: Ann, three years of age, discovers that when she plays with her clitoris she feels a very pleasant sensation. As she pursues this wonderful new discovery, her somewhat prudish mother discovers her and becomes horrified. Her mother spanks her, tells her she is a bad girl and forces her to wash her hands and go to bed. For Ann, there is a subsequent association of the functioning of the sexual glands and parts of the body with a feeling of tension. As she grows older and becomes interested in boys, her mother's attitude probably will make itself felt in her life again. All her efforts to meet and go out with boys will be accompanied by a certain feeling of dissatisfaction and disapproval. In other words, whenever her sexual glands are functioning normally, or when her body is being stimulated by them, there is an associated feeling of tension. During such times, the normal activity of the sexual glands and the sexual parts of the body may be disturbed.

Because breast development is dependent upon the normal functioning of these glands, it would not be unusual to find that Ann's breasts were very much delayed in their development. In fact, they might never develop fully until somehow this conditioning is altered.

Some Examples

Recently a 36-year old woman I had been counseling for several months reported to me that her breasts were enlarging rapidly not long after the resolution of several particularly disturbing childhood events. She is delighted that her breasts are "filling up" and developing a fullness and roundness that had not been there before.

Another case, Martha W., came into therapy when she was 15 years old. At the time of the first interview she showed a total absence of breast development and appeared below average in overall size. I found that her home environment was extremely disruptive. She suffered beatings, unfounded accusations, and excessive demands on her time and abilities. She then was removed from her family and stayed with relatives. Within six weeks her breasts had started developing and she had grown one inch in height. By the time she was sixteen years old — one year later — she had grown another five inches and her breasts were developing normally.

During the first treatment session of my study a 37-year old woman had a vivid recollection of her first period when she was 12 years old. She previously had reported in her questionnaire that she didn't begin menstruation until she was 15 or 16. She remembered she was wearing a bright yellow skirt and her period started unexpectedly (no one had told her anything about menstruation) while she was at school and she was covered with blood. "I was horribly frightened because I thought I might bleed to death." She was extremely embarrassed and walked all the way home from school saying to herself over and over, "I will not cry." She did not have another period until she was 16 years old and even then her embarrassment was extreme and she became very secretive about her monthly "problem."

This woman's emotional reactions had a decided effect on her menses and may have been a factor in retarding her breast growth. Upon completion of the 12-week treatment as a participant in the breast enlargement research, her breast size increased 1¼ inches.

Sixty-seven percent of the women in the study also said they were scared, shocked, or thought "it was horrible" when their periods first began. Over 70% reported experiencing "severe" discomfort, such as nausea, cramping, and headaches, when their menses began.

In 1969, Leslie LeCron, a clinical psychologist, reported in the *Journal of the American Society of Psychosomatic Dentistry and Medicine* that of 20 women he treated for breast enlargement, definite psychological factors were present which inhibited better breast development. These were usually remarks (which act as suggestions) belittling or making fun of their breasts or being told by relatives that they would never have nice-sized breasts. I found similar factors present with 87% of the women in my study, who reported feeling shamed or ridiculed by friends and relatives about their breasts. One participant said after completing the research, "I thought a lot about what happened during my adolescence. I never realized before how traumatic many things were for me."

Add to situations like this the influence of television, films, advertising, and magazines that repeatedly emphasize breasts primarily as objects of display, and it is no wonder that you might develop a chronic anxiety and concern for their size. If you can influence your body through your mind and interfere with normal breast growth, then you can undo any of these effects by reversing the process.

Are You Ready?

If you feel concern over the size of your breasts you can start changing all that today. If you are ready to increase your breast size, you have only to practice the exercises outlined in each chapter.

"Ready" means being able to accept as if it were true a mental picture of yourself with larger breasts.

"Ready" means a willingness to drop your present image of yourself and concede that you can have what you want. That may not be easy to do, but the rewards are tremendous because you can apply this same method to achieve other goals in your life: improved health, financial independence, satisfying personal relationships, career advancement, etc. The primary requirement is to accept that *you can have whatever you want.* I hope that you are not only "ready" but eager to do it.

"Ready" means working up the enthusiasm and excitement over the new prospects that await you.

"Ready" means surrendering to the process, giving up your doubts, and trusting your own mental faculties. Surrendering is not a matter of submitting to a competing force. Surrendering is being in neutral; it is non-resistance.

"Ready" means more than having faith that changes will occur. "Ready" means that you know that they are already on the way. And why not? You have nothing to lose, everything to gain, and these techniques can do you no harm. Certainly they are worth trying before deciding to use expensive and potentially dangerous surgical techniques.

Practice Exercise #4

Now get comfortable, put the book down, and allow your body to relax, as you did earlier. Then send these instructions to your mind:

> I accept my breast size as it is today as a temporary condition. I see myself relaxing daily and applying the new techniques. I see my instructions to my body being accepted by my subconscious mind and acted upon effectively.

Ready, go!

Chapter 5
LEFT AND RIGHT BRAIN

The brain is divided into two parts resembling the halves of a walnut, and these halves are called "left hemisphere" and "right hemisphere," or left brain and right brain. The left brain controls the right side of the body and the right brain controls the left side of the body. In a right-handed person the left brain is the dominant one and often is referred to as the thinking part of the brain. The left brain is verbal, rational and practical, describing, defining, drawing conclusions based on reasons and fact; it keeps track of time, and performs a number of other tidy and practical activities.

With the right brain we "see" things that may be imaginary — existing only in the mind's eye — or recall things that may be real. (Can you imagine your bedroom, for example?) When you use the right brain you understand metaphors, dream, create new combinations of ideas, and, when something is too complex to describe, you make gestures that communicate. The right side of the brain is intuitive, willing to suspend judgment, has little sense of time, is the artist, the dreamer, and usually is considered to be the subconscious. Thomas Blakeslee, author of *The Right Brain* suggests that a better choice of words would be "the non-verbal mind." However, for my purposes I will continue to use the term subconscious.

Two Ways of Knowing

Left and right terms are imbedded in our language and culture. The main divisions are between thinking and feeling, intellect and intuition. The key notion here is that there are two parallel ways of knowing. Sometimes the left half does not know what the right half is doing. While your brain gathers in sensory information, each half of the brain may be handling or processing that information in different ways. The job may be divided between the left and right brain, each handling the part best suited to its style. For instance, when you first learned to drive a

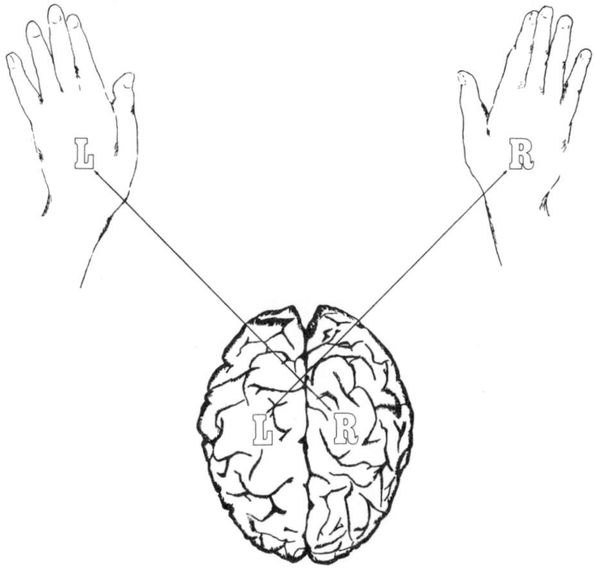

car, the left half of your brain inhibited the right half in order to get the job done quickly and because it is best suited to the task. Later, when your driving skill was mastered, the whole process became "subconscious" and automatic. The right hemisphere took over, freeing the left brain for other tasks.

I recently experienced great frustration in coping with this phenomenon when I attempted to describe a dream I had had. The dream was extremely vivid and I instinctively "knew" its meaning. When I started to explain the dream and what I "knew" to a friend, I found myself at a loss for the right words. I kept re-describing and re-explaining what I meant because it didn't sound right to me. What had seemed so clear and effortless in an instant became physically exhausting, as I shifted from my right brain's way of knowing to my left brain's way of functioning.

The Interfering Left Brain

Sometimes the two halves of the brain get in each other's way. For example: Did you ever feel like a dunce in your grade school art class? I did. No matter what I drew, it always came out a house with smoke rising from the chimney, one tree, the sun overhead and several lollipop looking flowers standing by a path. My art teacher's assessment? No creativity, no imagination. Result? I believed I couldn't draw even though I really loved to paint, crayon and make the pictures on paper. Because my dominant left brain, which had been highly developed during my grade school years in reading, writing, and arithmetic, felt it was better at the task of creating a picture, it jumped in to do the job. My less developed and "slower" right brain never had a chance to show its stuff. Often the dominant left brain will "take over" and hold the other half back.

Inhibiting the Left Brain

The nature of the task can influence which half will be in control and "take on a job" while holding back the other hemisphere. In her book, *Drawing on the Right Side of the Brain,* Betty Edwards creates a wonderful way for art students to inhibit the left brain and allow the right brain a chance to operate. She simply presents a picture upside down to her beginning art students and asks them to draw it. The left brain cannot make "sense" out of what it "sees" so it allows the right brain to take over for a while. Because the right brain is perfect for the task, drawing becomes easy and enjoyable. Her students' "before" and "after" drawings dramatically attest to the success of her method.

Enlarging your breasts is an ideal task for your right brain since it lacks a sense of time and is willing to suspend judgment as to whether or not enlarging your breasts now that you are beyond puberty makes any logical sense. While such information may be helpful, it is not necessary for you to "know" (left brain) about hormonal influences on your breast size, or the details about breast anatomy. The right brain is ideally suited for operating with visual images and will allow your body to respond appropriately. Like your nervous system, your right brain cannot tell the difference between what is imagined and what is real, as you already discovered when you imagined the lemon in Chapter one.

L-BRAIN

Left Brain Characteristics

Verbal: Using words to name, describe or define.

Analytic: Figuring things out, step by step.

Symbolic: Using a symbol to stand for something (like the plus sign stands for the process of addition).

Abstract: Using small bits of information to represent the entire thing.

Temporal: Keeping track of time sequences, one thing after another.

Rational: Drawing conclusions based on reason and fact.

Digital: Numbers and counting.

Logical: Drawing conclusions based on logic, one thing following another in a logical order (for example, a well-stated argument).

Linear: Thinking in terms of linked ideas, one thought directly following another, often leading to a convergent conclusion.

R-BRAIN

Right Brain Characteristics

Non-verbal: Being aware of things, but having minimal connections with words.

Synthetic: Putting things together to form wholes.

Concrete: Relating to things as they are at the present moment.

Analogic: Seeing likenesses between things, understanding metaphors.

Non-Temporal: Lacking a sense of time.

Non-Rational: Not requiring a basis of reason or fact, willingness to suspend judgment. Sometimes emotional.

Spatial: Knowing where things are in relation to other things and how parts go together to form a whole.

Intuitive: Making leaps of insight often based on incomplete patterns, hunches, fears, or visual images.

Wholistic: Seeing whole things all at once, perceiving the over-all patterns and structures often leading to divergent conclusions.

*Taken from Edwards, *Drawing on the Right Side of the Brain.* NY: J.P. Tarcher, 1979.

Practice Exercise #5

> Picture the two halves of your brain, left and right, much as they are depicted in the drawing. Right now close your eyes, take a few deep breaths, relax and image the left side in a blue color and the right side in a red color.
>
> Now picture in your mind the connections from your left brain to the right side of your body. Imagine them any way that you wish — as tubes, wires, electrical currents or whatever. Picture the blue pathways going from your left brain to every portion and part of the right side of your body. Good, now shift to the other side. Imagine red connections between your right brain and the left side of your body. Wonderful, now take a deep breath and open your eyes.

By doing the preceding exercise you will be able to call forth an image of what I'm describing rather than to think about it in words.

Practice Exercise #6

Since enlarging your breasts with your mind is primarily a right brain function, it is important to keep the left brain out of it. So for your purposes I want you now to direct your attention to the right side of your brain.

> Repeat the mental exercise above and this time imagine the red connections going from your right brain and concentrating in the area of your breasts. Imagine the red color growing brighter and more intense. The brighter and stronger it gets the more it influences your breasts to grow larger. Pretend the red color is your blood pulsating into your breasts and bringing nourishment to all the cells of your breast. Imagine the fat and glandular cells not only enlarging, but dividing and multiplying as well. Good, now take a deep breath and open your eyes.

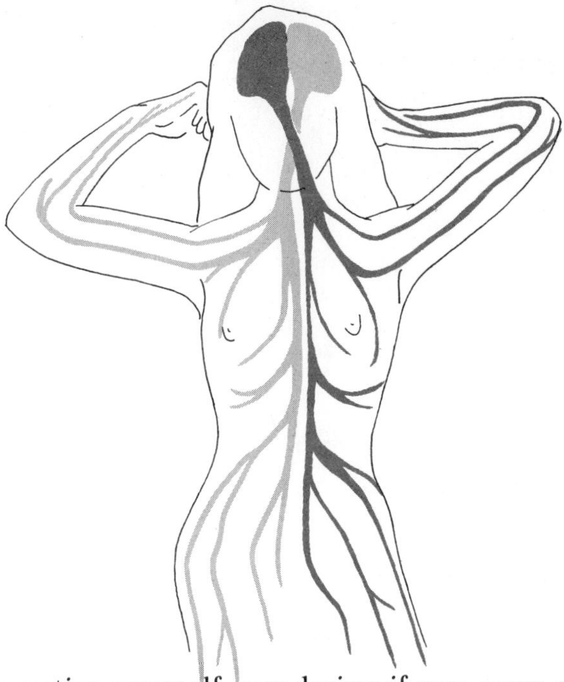

Did you notice yourself wondering if you were doing this exercise "right"? Then you just experienced your analytical and critical thinking left brain.

The problem is that the dominant left brain is very speedy and is prone to rushing in to take over a job that it is not good at accomplishing. Thus you set up a conflict between your thoughts and your imagination. To eliminate this possibility, allow yourself to enter into a deeply relaxed state, just as you did in Chapter one, in order to bring all efforts of the left brain to a minimum.

You Have Done It Before

Deep relaxation is easy to do because you have been in this pleasantly relaxed state naturally hundreds of times. You have been doing this every day of your life. You're already an expert at it.

Remember being so engrossed in a book that you simply did not hear your name being called, although it was quite audible? The material in the book was so interesting that your mind had "turned off" most of its attention to the rest of the world. Whenever you daydream, watch a movie, watch TV, spend long hours driving, or get lost in listening to a particular piece of music, you are screening out other sensory information to your left brain. You are focusing on only one set of stimuli which automatically allows your right brain to function.

Daydreaming, being engrossed in a book, watching TV or a movie are all similar: you are concentrating passively on thought patterns as they pass through your mind. In each case very little effort was needed to achieve this state of mind. The thought processes merely were allowed to flow. You now are going to use the same process here only now you will be doing it on purpose.

Your senses are accosted daily by a vast array of stimuli: the weather, people, lights, noises, food, clothing, colors. Many of these things are irritating to you or not essential to what you are doing at the moment, so you automatically screen them out of your conscious thinking. You don't give them your attention because to do so would bring chaos into your life. Even so, you're coping with more sensations than you need. The first step is to quiet your mind, eliminate the non-essential sensations. In this way you can focus your mind and concentrate all its power on achieving your desired breast size.

Practice Exercise #7

Sit or lie down comfortably. Take a deep breath and, as you relax, tell yourself that any movement or sound around you helps you to relax even more. Now close your eyes and imagine all your old thoughts about not being able to affect your body with your mind being carried off in a helium-filled balloon. Imagine the balloon, filled with your fears and doubts about your success, getting smaller and smaller as it goes farther and farther away, until finally the balloon is almost gone. Now you can let your conscious (left brain) thoughts go wherever you want them to. You can even go to sleep if you want.

Chapter 6
RELAXATION

The natural breast enlargement process encourages you to make use of your natural suggestibility, an ability that you already possess. There is no strain, no concentration and no will power required. In fact, if you use will power or strain to concentrate, you actually may hamper the ability of your mind to bring about the changes you desire. Suppose I offered you $5,000 to increase your breast size by using will power and concentration. Do you think you'd ever collect the money? No matter how hard you tried or how much effort you put into it, your labors would be in vain. Called the "law of reverse effect," it works like this: the harder you TRY, the more you believe you can't succeed.

Instead of trying hard by conscious effort and telling yourself all the things you're doing wrong, simply relax the strain and use that wonderful creative imagination of yours to picture yourself in a comfortable chair or bed and imagine yourself relaxing.

When using your imagination, you may notice that you will tend to fall into one of two main categories of people: you are a "visualizer" or a "senser." Visualizers see images and sensers feel or even hear them. Each type has its advantages so simply accept your imagination the way it is.

The First Step

The first step to increasing your breasts is a relaxing process that helps to clear your mental channels by reducing stress and decreasing nervousness so that your breast enlargement messages can get through.

Pick a time and place where you will not be disturbed, perhaps in the evening before going to bed or when you awaken in the morning.

If possible, shut out any loud noises, bright lights, harsh odors, or any other uncomfortable sensation that you might allow to have an effect on you. The best idea is to suggest to yourself that all these factors help you to relax more and more. Loosen any tight clothing. Take off your shoes. Undo. Unsnap. Unzip.

Practice Exercise #8

First of all, get to know what a relaxed muscle is. Tense your jaw by biting down on your teeth. Then let your jaw go slack. Do the same with your hands, arms, or legs. Or pick out a tense spot on your body and make it tighter and more tense. (Good places to look for tenseness are the back of your neck, your shoulders or your chest.) Make this spot as tight as you can, the tighter the better. Now hold it for a count of three — don't let go — 1 - 2 - 3. Now let go completely. Breathe. Now you're ready to read on.

Take a deep breath and let it out slowly. Feel your whole body go flat as you let the air out like a limp balloon. Now close your eyes. Use the moment you close your eyes as a signal that you have shut out the world from your thoughts. Take about ten seconds to do this. Your primary goal is to bring about a relaxed state of your mind and your body.

Do this exercise in either a sitting or a lying position. The aim is to create an ideal situation in which your mind can drift on its own without effort or concentration and become a clear channel for your breast enlargement images. You can use any method that works for you. Here are some examples to get you started.

Practice Exercise #9

After you have closed your eyes, consciously "let go" the various muscle groups of your body as much as you can, like you did a few moments ago. Just pay attention to the various parts of your body and let go a little. You may find that you can always voluntarily relax to some degree. Stop frowning and let your forehead relax. Ease up a little in the tension in your jaws. Let your hands, your arms, your shoulders, and your legs become more relaxed than they are right now. Take about five minutes to do this. Then don't pay attention anymore to your muscles. This is as far as you need go in using your conscious control. From here on, relax more and more by using your wonderful ability to pretend and you will easily bring about a relaxed condition. In other words, you are going to allow your non-verbal right brain to automatically reach these goals for you.

Practice Exercise #10

In your mind's eye see yourself stretched out on your bed and picture your body as it would look if it was made of lumps of lead. See yourself lying there with two very heavy leaden legs. Notice how these leaden legs sink farther and farther down into the mattress. Now imagine your arms and hands made of lumps of lead. Your arms and hands are very, very heavy and they are sinking down into the bed. In fact, you notice the tremendous pressure that they exert against the bed. Now in your mind's eye, see a friend coming into the room and attempting to lift your heavy leaden legs. She takes hold of your foot and tries to lift it, but it's too heavy — she can't do it. Now she takes hold of your arm and tries to lift it, but it weighs too much — she can't lift your arm. Now she tries to lift you around your neck but once again you are as heavy as concrete and she is unable to lift you and you sink deeper and deeper into the bed.

Practice Exercise #11

Imagine that your body is like a puppet on a string. Your hands are tied to your wrists by loose strings. Your forearm is connected loosely by a string to your upper arm. Your upper arm is connected very loosely by a string to your shoulders. Your feet, calves, thighs, everything in your whole body is connected together with a very loose limp string. Your neck consists of one very, very limp string.

The strings that control your jaw and hold your lips together have slackened and stretched to such an extent that your chin has dropped down against your chest. All the different strings that connected the various parts of the body are loose and limp and your body is sprawled loosely across the bed, completely relaxed.

Practice Exercise #12

Now again use your "let's make believe" imagination. See your body as a bunch of inflated rubber balloons. You have two valves in your feet and, in your mind's eye, you open the valve and the air begins to escape from your legs. Your legs begin to collapse and continue to collapse until they consist only of deflated rubber tubes. And they lie flat against the bed. Next you open a valve in your chest and as the air begins to escape your entire abdomen and chest begin to collapse limply against the bed. Continue to let the air out of your arms, your head, and your neck.

Practice Exercise #13

This may be the easiest and most relaxing image of all. Recall a time and place when you felt relaxed and at peace with the world. If you can't recall one, make one up. It may have been a place in the mountains or a summer day at the beach or a quiet relaxing time somewhere in your own home. Remember all the little incidental things, what sounds were present, what you saw. Recall the smells and the texture of the things around you.

The more vividly you are able to recall the specific details and picture them to yourself the more successful you will be when you use the same procedure to enlarge your breasts.

You have the key. Hang on to it. Practice it. Use it.

The more you use this key the more successful you will be at relaxing immediately whenever you want.

You are now at the stage where you are mastering the art of relaxation. The suggestions you give yourself while relaxed are helping to deepen your powers of relaxation.

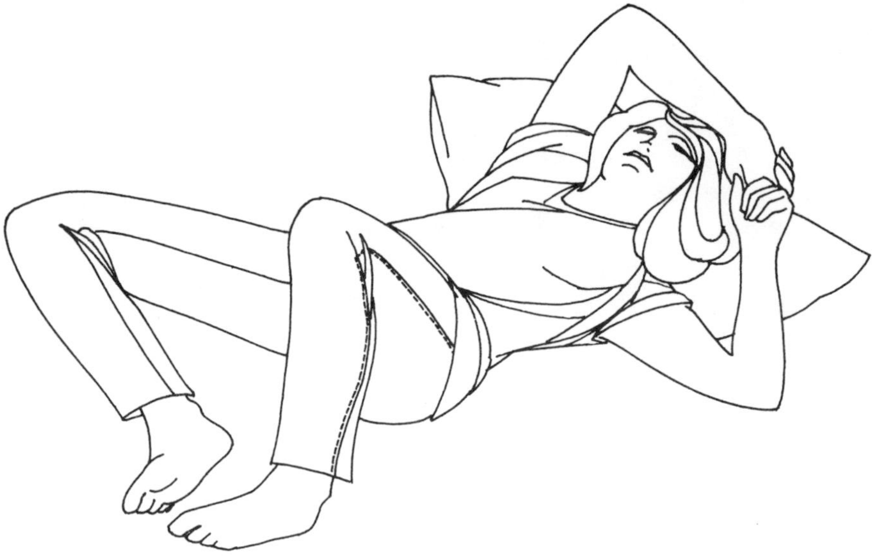

Other Techniques to Quiet Your Mind

Another effective technique to quiet your mind is to pretend you're in a light gray cloud. Your thoughts cannot enter the cloud. They cannot penetrate through to you.

Surround yourself with this thought protection.

If you find the cloud doesn't work for you, build an imaginary room around yourself with light gray walls, floor and ceiling.

Remember, don't make this into a big effort to keep thoughts out. That is the opposite of being relaxed. Instead, watch your thoughts come and go and soon they will leave you altogether.

For a really stubborn case there is one more useful technique: Pretend you are sitting in a quiet room with a blackboard in front of you. On it are the numbers from one through ten. If a thought enters your mind to disturb you, you mentally erase the number ten. If it happens again, you "get up" and erase the number nine telling yourself that when you finally erase number one, your mind will be a clean slate and you'll be deeply relaxed.

How Will You Know if You're Relaxed?

Each person will feel something different. When you're completely relaxed you may feel as if you are floating, or you may feel quite heavy. Another time you may feel as though parts of your body have disappeared or you may feel a gentle rocking motion. You may not feel any change at all. Obviously no particular way of feeling is better than any other. The "correct" feeling is simply the one you are having at the time. If you are doing the exercise, you are doing it right.

If you have followed your relaxation suggestions you are relaxed whether you feel differently or not.

Be aware that you can hinder your progress into deep relaxation by allowing your analytical and critical left brain to get into the act. Some thoughts you may notice that can cause you to doubt:

"I wonder if I'm doing this right."	You are.
"I wonder if it's working."	It is.
"Did I use the right picture?"	You did.

Whenever you have these critical thoughts, dismiss them from your mind by telling yourself you are doing it right. You are doing it effectively. Your old way was to doubt, now you're finding a new way. Your only purpose here is to relax and confidently repeat to yourself, "When I'm relaxed enough, I'll be able to give myself the breast enlargement suggestions that work."

Chapter 7
VISUALIZATION

One of the marvelous abilities of the right brain is visualization or seeing an imaginary picture with "your mind's eye." The brain is able to conjure up an image and then "work" at it, "seeing" it as if it is "really there." I am describing the awesome power of your imagination. Don't be tempted to say you "have no imagination." When it comes right down to it everyone has a pretty good imagination or they would never *worry* about anything.

Remember the examples presented in Chapter one? Perhaps you prayed for a healthy strong body or you wanted to have a loved one respond to you in a particular way. As you prayed, you held certain pictures in your mind (whether you realized it or not) of how you wanted your prayer to be answered. When those pictures were "real," you "knew" your prayers had been answered.

When you wanted a new car, you thought about the model you wanted, what color you wanted, how much mileage you would get. You pictured your needs, (will the whole family fit in the car, or is it just for me) and after you checked around for the best price, you bought one.

When you told yourself that something terrible was going to happen, you first had a "funny" feeling that you couldn't logically explain. Then you worried and fretted about what it might be. You allowed your mind to dwell on every negative outcome you could possibly imagine. Then, when something happened that you hadn't expected to occur, you "knew" that was the terrible thing that you were expecting. (Not only is your subconscious amenable to reason, it is amenable to lack of reason, too.)

These are all examples of your imagination at work. If you have ever worried, prayed, talked to yourself, or played "make believe," then you already "know" how to enlarge your breasts.

Suggestibility

Using your imagination to relax and enlarge your breasts is possible because all human beings are suggestible. We are all susceptible to being influenced in varying degrees, either by ourselves or by another person. For instance, have you ever seen someone else yawn and found yourself yawning involuntarily, even against your most strenuous efforts? Or noticed your foot tapping unconsciously to the beat of exciting music? Perhaps you found yourself laughing for no other reason than that other people around you were laughing. These are examples of simple non-verbal suggestions to which you automatically responded.

The wonderful gift of *suggestibility* is a key factor in changing your breasts by reprogramming your mind. Although your dream of developing larger breasts may be different from someone else's, your mind can work for you in an individual way to bring about the changes you desire.

Developing your suggestibility is done with mental images and *pretending* that what you imagine is real.

Visualizing and pretending "as if" are important elements both in relaxing your mind and body and in increasing the size and shape of your breasts.

How Does Visualization Work?

You apply plain common sense in a very practical way. Everything you want starts with a mental image. If you want a house, you visualize the type of building you want, with the floor plan, landscaping and maybe the furniture. Your mental imagery is then projected onto paper in the form of a sketch, then a design, then blueprints and specifications and then finally it is built.

The easiest way to formulate an idea is to visualize it. Indeed, that is the *only* way ideas are formed. You first learn to think in pictures, not words. Out of necessity you had to learn the appropriate words to describe your pictures to others. What you form in your imagination is as real as any part of your body.

A woman in my breast enlargement study used her ability to pretend by imaging "workers stacking healthy fat packages onto flatbed trucks parked on my thighs. The workers trucked the packages up to my chest where fat masons stacked them on my breasts." Since she desired to have the upper portion of her breasts filled in, she pretended "as if" the fat packages were stacked there. She increased her breast size by one and one-half inches.

The degree to which you will be successful with the Natural Breast Enlargement program is dependent on how you apply the "As If" principle. The "As If" principle states that you accept the suggestions and images you give yourself "as if" they were true. Of course you will be giving yourself true suggestions, but if you think they won't work, they won't. If you know they will work, they will. Accept your own suggestions as if they are an accomplished fact, and accomplished they will be.

Practice Exercise #14

Start practicing to accept your own suggestions "as if" they were true right now. Read these instructions, then put the book aside and begin.

> First I want you to hold your arms out parallel in front of you, with your palms facing each other just a few inches apart. Keep your thumbs up. Close your eyes. Now turn on that wonderful creative imagination of yours. Visualize a heavy weight over your left wrist — perhaps a shopping bag full of heavy canned goods. Imagine that it is very, very heavy. At the same time, pretend a balloon filled with helium is attached to your right wrist with a string. It pulls your wrists upward. You haven't completed this exercise until you can picture and "feel" the heavy weight of the shopping bag pulling your right arm upward. When you are sure that you have pictured it as though it were true, open your eyes.

If you were able to visualize this exercise "as if" it were true — that is, if you pretended that the bag and the balloon were really there — when you opened your eyes you probably found that your left arm was lower than your right arm.

For some of you, it may have been only a slight difference. For others, the left arm may have been slanted downward very sharply toward the floor and the right arm raised in an angle toward the ceiling, with perhaps a substantial distance between the palms. Even if your palms were only an inch apart vertically, you have demonstrated that you have the power to visualize "as if it were true."

If you were not satisfied with the movement, practice it again and do it until you see good results. Don't consciously think about moving your arms. Rather, use your conscious mind to pretend the heavy weight and the balloon. Forget about your arms. Let your subsconscious mind do all the rest. The ability to pretend is vital to programming your subconscious mind to enlarge your breasts.

Chapter 8

DEVELOPING YOUR PERSONAL PLAN

Everyday happenings were at one time mental images and thoughts held long enough and ardently enough that they became motivating forces in your subconscious mind.

"I want to be a Cellist."

"I'm going for my Ph.D. in Anthropology."

"I'm hoping to get my real estate license."

If you were just mouthing the words and didn't achieve your goal, then what you were demonstrating was an ability to *talk* about your dreams not achieve them. If you really do not think you have the ability to become a cellist, anthropologist, or realtor, and just like to talk about it, is it likely that you will be successful in achieving your goal? No. You need to picture your results as though they have already occurred.

Now that you're familiar with the ingredients basic to the Natural Breast Enlargement program, you need to develop a plan to insure your success. Your personal plan consists of:

1. YOUR GOAL — a clear vision of how you want to look.
2. ACCEPTANCE — the elimination of negative suggestions.
3. TRUST — cancelling out the negative critical factor.
4. PRACTICE — using "make believe" daily to achieve the results you want.

Your Goal

Enlarging your breasts starts with a picture held in your imagination of how you want your breasts to look. Your present image of your breasts grew out of many years of interpretations and evaluations of yourself based on your past "experiences." Now you are to use the same method to enlarge your breasts that was used to inhibit their growth.

Is it important to go over, in your mind, exactly the way you want your breasts to look? Yes! Picture them vividly. You may have had trouble visualizing in the past and may be saying "but I can't picture a thing." If so, find a photograph in a magazine of a woman who approximates your body size and type. Such pictures are readily located in ads for bathing suits. If you prefer, use a photo of a nude woman. Your feelings may change as you go along. Several women I worked with told me that they preferred pictures of women with their breasts covered because they were not comfortable with nudity. One such woman later switched to using a photo of a nude woman. I asked her why she had changed and she told me that she no longer felt embarrassed looking at the naked model.

Once you have a photo that pleases you, use a head shot of yourself from either a snapshot or a new photograph and place this photo of your head on the body of the picture that you have chosen. Be sure the two pictures are in proper proportion to each other. The photo will help you focus more vividly on how *you* want to look. Remember to follow your own instincts and ideas on how you want to look — not the ideas of how someone else might want you to appear.

Now, incorporate as many of your senses as possible.

Touch. Imagine your breasts larger and how they feel to your touch.

Smell. Imagine the aroma of your favorite perfume or body lotion which you have just used on your breasts and enjoy its fragrance.

Hearing. Imagine the surprise and amazement of other people and what they are saying about your successfully enlarging your breasts. Be sure to imagine people who like you and who will encourage your efforts.

Emotions. Emotions are *very* important. Use your wonderful ability to pretend how confident you will *feel* when your breasts are as large or as shapely as you want them to be. Feel the emotional pleasure, joy and pride you will experience from the extra attention given to your full breasts.

Have you created a clear picture of how you want to look? If you have, get ready to put the book down and have some fun. You're about to pretend that you have larger breasts.

Practice Exercise #15

> Picture a calendar date three to six months from now. Pretend your goal is reached — See it — Sense it — Take it all in — Enjoy it — Create the details — Act it out in your mind.

The main thing to remember is that once your subconscious is presented with a picture of how you want your breasts to look and *accepts* it, it begins to make it happen.

Two women who participated in my study wanted to equalize the size of each breast. The first woman was 31-years old, married, had two children and imagined a scale to balance the proportions of each breast. At the end of the study her left breast increased in size and her right breast decreased in size. She had an overall increase of breast measurement of 2 inches.

The other participant was single, 24-years old, and a nursing student. She wanted to increase the size of her left breast, which was one-half the size of her right breast. She used a "fantastic journey" type of imagery. She imagined a heavy supply of blood carrying large amounts of androgens and estrogens to her left breast. She also pictured "sub-cutaneous fat being deposited in the left breast to add inches and fullness." She was successful with her "make-believe" and achieved 3/4 inch overall increase in her breast measurement. The change in size and shape of her breasts was very noticeable to other women in her group who complimented her on her achievement. The point to be made here is that the idea and thoughts are real and will one day appear in your objective world, if you persist with your mental imaging.

Acceptance

Now you are ready for the next step: accept reaching your goal of larger breasts. That may sound silly, since you wouldn't picture what you want and then have to *convince* yourself that it's acceptable when you reach your goal. The problem of acceptance isn't silly though. People who don't accept their own goals are constantly programming themselves not to act. If you say you want larger breasts and also believe it doesn't matter if you have larger breasts, then your automatic mind records both messages and says "does not compute." Each thought cancels out the other.

For example, a woman came to me to quit smoking. She said that every time she decided to give it up she found herself smoking more. Upon questioning, I discovered she had a horror of gaining weight, even just a few pounds. Every time she tried to imagine herself as a non-smoker (a positive image) she also experienced intense feelings of fear, doubt, and anxiety. She became afraid of giving up her habit because she did not believe such a thing could happen without putting her in some kind of danger. Thus she not only had not been able to stop smoking, but she found herself smoking more because it reduced her intense fears and anxiety.

A negative feeling that was frequently reported to me by the women I have seen for breast enlargement was the hot flush of embarrassment they felt when anyone called attention to their breasts. One notion many of the women believed was that large-breasted girls were considered "easy." This interpretation apparently was made because large-breasted girls seemed to receive so much attention from the boys.

The purpose of uncovering your own unwanted thoughts and feelings is to escape their inevitability. Thus you become free to choose whether or not you want to keep them and their effects on your life.

Eliminate Unwanted Suggestions

Right now I want you to check out your own feelings and thoughts to see if you have any negative suggestions about your having larger breasts left over from past experiences. Here is an extremely important step in using your mind to enlarge your breasts and one that is left out of most other self-help books. You need to be aware of the negatives in order to steer clear of them.

To give new suggestions without first removing old contradictory suggestions would create a state of anxiety and conflict within you, and would very possibly keep your from reaching your goal.

After you have located an early negative experience in your memory, change it around to suit you. For instance, maybe someone made fun of your breasts or ridiculed you in some way because of them. Erase this negative suggestion to yourself by changing the situation. See that same person complimenting you. Turn the memory into a **win** for yourself! You cannot change the actual event, but you can at least alter your emotional reaction to it.

Once you have become conscious of a fear, doubt or other negative thought, you also are free to choose to eliminate it from your life. Here's an effective way to rid yourself of any fear that might be holding you back from having the breast size you want.

WHAT IS THE WORST POSSIBLE THING THAT COULD HAPPEN WHEN YOU HAVE LARGER BREASTS?

Really visualize it. Locate the source of your fear by identifying the first time you felt it or thought it. Then re-live it in your imagination. Unspecific fears are the most destructive. As soon as you have a clear view of what you fear, the fear itself usually diminishes. See how irrelevant it is for you today. You're much older, wiser, more competent than you were when you first had the fear. It no longer applies to you in your life today. It is irrelevant.

File it under "garbage."

Now do your positive reprogramming. Repeat the following affirmation:

> Negative thoughts about having larger breasts no longer influence me. I deserve larger breasts and that's what I want! Positive thoughts now bring me the results I desire.

Practice Exercise #16

Now keeping these things in mind, place yourself in a deep state of relaxation as you learned to do earlier.

> Create a picture of your present self in your mind. Now let it disappear and create another image of yourself as you ultimately want your breasts to look and as they will look when you succeed. While you mentally gaze at the new you, imagine in as much detail as you possibly can what it will feel like to have larger, fuller breasts. How will you feel when you put on your clothes? When you are drying yourself after a bath? Walking around a pool or a beach in your bathing suit?
>
> Take your time and "feel" all these scenes in your mind. Go through your senses, one at a time, as described earlier. How will your attitude toward yourself change as the result of achieving your goal? What does that feel like?
>
> Now envision your breasts growing as you rest comfortably, once or twice a day, using this program. Use whatever affirmative suggestions that you have previously chosen.

As you progress with your program your total mental state about your breasts will improve and this improvement, in turn, will contribute to successfully enlarging your breasts. Now you know why "positive thinking" alone cannot be used effectively to enlarge your breasts. The Natural Breast Enlargement program goes beyond positive thinking by alerting you to your negative thoughts so that you can change them. Your must free yourself of the unwanted body images and feelings left over from long ago.

Trust

You are now on your way to having the breast size that you have always wanted.

What was your reaction when you read that sentence? Did you start rejecting the "possibility" of truth in that simple statement? Did your conditioned mind automatically say, "Not me,".

"No way," "Oh Yeah?," "Is she kidding?." "It might work for someone else, but not for me."

Give up SELF-LIMITATION. Reject your doubts. If you persist "knowing" the program won't work, your subconscious right brain will take you at your word and follow your orders. "Hey, stop the process! The Boss doesn't want to enlarge her breasts." Accept the program by "knowing" that it will work for you.

Learn to TRUST your creative right brain to do its work and avoid "jamming it" by becoming too concerned or too anxious as to whether it will work or not, or by attempting to force it by too much conscious effort. If you are following the instructions you'll find success. You "let it" work, rather than "make it" work. Your trust is important because your creative right brain operates below the level of consciousness, and you cannot "know" what is going on beneath the surface.

Don't wait until you have "proof" your breasts enlarged to *believe* they are enlarging. Pretend as if they already are larger and you will be successful. There is no "can" or "can't" involved here. The question is whether you want larger breasts or don't want them. Your goal is something you want to reach, so reach it and you will.

Until you see definite results, I suggest that you tell as few people as possible (none is best) that you are using these techniques to enlarge your breasts. You need time to strengthen your own positive suggestions before you subject yourself and your progress to those who have not yet accepted these ideas. Check with your mate and see if he will be comfortable with your having larger breasts. Three women dropped out of my study because their husbands or boyfriends did not like the idea of them having larger breasts.

If you are hearing negative comments from your mate, friends, co-workers or others you will need to strengthen your positive programming. You do this three ways:

1. You reinforce your insulation against negative suggestions from the outside using the techniques described above.
2. You strengthen your own positive suggestions for goal attainment with "I am" affirmations.
3. You insure your success by programming yourself to fight for goal attainment. "I am not affected by the 'failure' thoughts of others. Negativity bounces off me. Positivity I accept."

Imagining others praising you or marveling at your success has the function of reinforcing the effect you are programming. Visualizing yourself as the center of positive attention is a powerful reward for your subconscious. Don't let others' reactions or lack of reaction discourage you!

Repeat to yourself the following affirmation:

> I accept my goal of larger breasts as natural and right for me. I desire it. I am being myself. I am expressing my true nature. I am for larger breasts. I have them!

Practice

The Natural Breast Enlargement program requires that you be a self-starter. Be nice to *you* and **make an appointment** with yourself to relax and pretend daily. Tell yourself there are no exceptions to using the program daily. Exceptions are a way the negative parts of you weaken your resolve and dilute your decision to reach your goal. I've included a progress chart at the back of the book so you can keep track of each session. It will be easy to remember your appointments to relax, because these periods are healthful, energizing, and restorative. Once you begin to practice relaxing regularly, your ability to relax quickly increases with every session.

Realize that the only way that you can experience the benefits from using your mind to enlarge your breasts is by actually using the suggestions consistently over a period of time. When researched, this program ran three months, so plan on at least that amount of time.

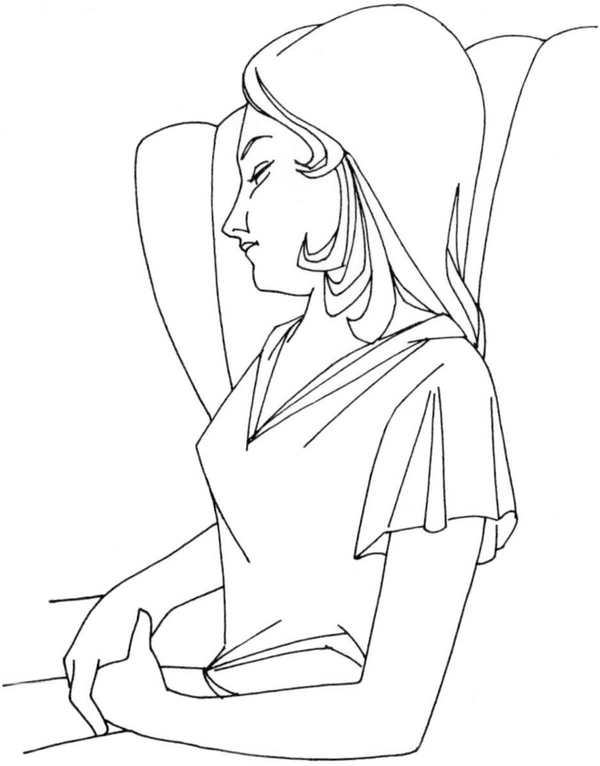

When you use Natural Breast Enlargement techniques, plan on twenty to thirty minutes for each session. Set aside any time of the day that is convenient for you, even if it's in the middle of the night. This is your program, right? Each subsequent time you use Natural Breast Enlargement you will notice that you relax more deeply in a shorter period of time and automatically remember the suggestions. When you find this happening give yourself a key word or phrase that allows you to relax quickly. My favorite word is "Relax." I say it to myself as I take a deep breath and then slowly let it out. By the time I've exhaled I'm very deeply relaxed. Use whatever works best for you. The key word or thought instantly reminds your wonderful creative right brain of the whole process of being relaxed and PRESTO, you're relaxed and ready to give yourself your breast enlargement suggestions.

Chapter 9

THE NATURAL BREAST ENLARGEMENT PROGRAM

The following series of suggestions is presented to enable you to reach your goal of enlarging your breasts. Plan on using the suggestions daily until you achieve the results you want. Then use them occasionally to maintain your increase in breast size if you wish. Most women notice some increase within four to twelve weeks. Most of the women in my study noticed a moderate increase within the first four weeks. The most rapid increase seems to occur during the second month.

If you have not enlarged your breasts to the degree you want by the end of the third month, I suggest you write a new monologue and use it for an indefinite period of time until your breasts have developed to the size you desire. Be sure to develop detailed instructions and include all your senses and emotions for the changes you desire. You may also wish to review Chapter eight, just in case there are some contradictory negative suggestions from the past still affecting you.

It is essential that you disregard past failures with other breast enlargement devices. This is the time — right now — to tear up old score cards and start afresh. Your motivation and interest should be at a peak; your expectations, the greatest. Be confident that you are on the threshold of a new time of self-mastery.

You're Unique

Expect gradual progress weekly with the largest amount of increase coinciding monthly with your menstrual cycle. DO NOT COMPARE your results with anyone else's. You're unique and you might increase your breast size in a few weeks, whereas it might take someone else two to three months. Where your breasts add inches or fullness may differ completely from where another woman's breasts add inches or fullness. Some of the women in my study showed breast increases on the upper inside portion (toward your heart) of their breasts, while on others the increase was measurable on the outer portion of the breast (toward your arm). Some women had an even increase all around their breasts, and others achieved a balancing effect. The amount and type of breast enlargement varies according to your own desires, needs and expectations of what you consider adequate development. You may be satisfied with just firming up, while another woman may want to increase her cup-size.

Because these suggestions are based on your own directions, you can read them to yourself or have a friend read them to you.

Make a Tape

Recording the suggestions is a very effective device to speed you on your way to deep relaxation. With a recording you can relax and eliminate distractions. A taped recording removes the possibility of feeling self-conscious if someone is reading the suggestions to you. Even if others are around, by using a recording you can add headphones or earphones so you can keep the playback private. You can either make your own recording, or have the suggestions recorded by a friend.

You may want to hear a male voice giving you the suggestions to enlarge your breasts. One woman in my study who had minimal increase in breast size said she felt she would have enlarged her breasts if a man's voice had been used. She was an exception, however, since the remaining women said they would have felt very uncomfortable hearing a male voice and probably wouldn't have volunteered to do the research. I feel their concern was associated more with the type of breast enlargement suggestion they thought a man would prepare rather than actually hearing a male voice. As Ayalah and Weinstock point out in their book *Breasts,* "Often a woman's experience of her breasts is directly influenced by her experiences with men and by men's attitudes and feelings about women's breasts." As long as the suggestions are sensitive to *your* needs and desires I don't feel it makes any difference.

If you make your own recording, pause during the taping so that you will have plenty of time to follow the directions as you listen to it. You can experiment with the monologue I present here or make up your own. The recording provides you with a playback of your own directions in your own voice. After a few weeks you can change the monologues if you desire, to make it more interesting.

One of the best times to listen to your tape is just before going to bed. The twilight state just before you drift off to sleep is perfect for relaxing. You do not have to be completely awake because your suggestions are working even in this semi-awake state. If you find yourself going deeply asleep, then use the tape one hour earlier. You can also listen to the tape any other time of day if bedtime is not convenient.

Now Get Ready To Relax

1. Find a comfortable place where you can feel relaxed. For most people, this will be a reclining position, but, if you tend to fall asleep very easily, a sitting position may be preferable. While it is possible to experience an induction standing up or in any other position, lying down will probably be the most comfortable for you at this stage.

2. Before sitting or lying down, make sure you have no obligations for the next thirty minutes. Any concerns about parking meters which might run overtime, phone calls you may be expecting or oven timers due to go off soon will serve as significant distractions.

3. Loosen your clothing. Go to the bathroom before you begin if you think it might interfere later.

4. REMEMBER, ABOVE ALL, DO NOT EVALUATE YOUR PROGRESS, THE SUGGESTIONS THEMSELVES, OR ANYTHING ELSE THAT COMES TO MIND DURING THE PROCESS.

5. Now turn on your tape or have a friend read the suggestions to you.

NATURAL BREAST ENLARGEMENT SUGGESTIONS

Make yourself as comfortable as possible. During the next few minutes you will relax completely. The only important thing right now is to completely relax your body, mind and emotions. The only thing that will be required of you is to relax and let go. You effortlessly listen and respond to the directions. Though you think you have experienced relaxation before, now you will really know complete relaxation.

First, fill your lungs with air. Slowly expand your chest and abdominal muscles and hold your breath. Feel the tension. Now slowly exhale the air from your lungs. Feel the tension begin to disappear.

In the next few moments, you will relax every muscle in your body, relaxing each muscle group effortlessly, naturally and easily. You will tense a muscle group and then relax it slowly. In between each tensing and relaxation exercise, take a deep breath, effortlessly and easily, exhaling the air slowly from your lungs, achieving a relaxation that you've never experienced before. The only important thing right now is to completely relax your mind, your body, and your emotions. The only thing required of you is to relax and let go. You effortlessly listen and respond to the directions, effortlessly and easily let go . . . let go . . . and relax.

As if by automatic response, you will first tense and then relax the various muscle groups in your body. These muscles will be held under tension until I count to three, then slowly release them. Focus now . . . center your attention on your toes. Curl your toes tightly away from your face and hold it until I count to three. Good . . . 1 . . . 2 . . . 3. Relax and let go. Breathe deeply . . . breathe in deeply and relax more as your exhale. Fine. Now, curl your toes tightly toward your face. Tighter, tighter. Hold it . . . 1 . . . 2 . . . 3 . . . relax and let go. Breathe in deeply and exhale as you let your relaxation become complete. Good. Now create tension in the calves of your legs. Tense them tightly, hold it . . . 1 . . . 2 . . . 3 . . . Relax and let go. Wonderful. Now another deep breath. All the way in . . . let go . . . and relax. Now center your mind on the muscles in your thighs, from your knees to your hips. Tighten them. Tense . . . hold it . . . 1 . . . 2 . . . 3. Relax and let go. Fine. Breathe all the way in and all the way out. Notice the relaxation. Feel the blood flowing freely through the arteries and veins of your legs and feet. You are letting go. Good. Now focus your attention on your face and head. Wrinkle your brow . . . tighten your closed eyes . . . push your tongue against the roof of your mouth. Hold it tightly. 1 . . . 2 . . . 3. Relax and let go. Gently. Excellent. Gently fill your lungs with air and now let it go. Now pull your chin against your chest. Down tight, tighter. Hold it . . . 1 . . . 2 . . . 3. Relax and let go. Let your head shift effortlessly back into relaxation. Wonderful. Breathe in gently and softly exhale. Feel the relaxation in your head, your neck and your legs. Next, make your hands into fists and tense your arms all the way to the shoulders. Good. Tighter, tighter. 1 . . . 2 . . . 3. Relax and let go. Fine. Fill your lungs now and gently let the air out. Notice the pleasant and calm feeling that you're beginning to experience throughout your body. Now, arch your back and pull your shoulders together. Pull tightly. Hold it. 1 . . . 2 . . . 3. Relax and let go. Good. Another gentle deep breath and let it out gently. Pull your abdomen all the way in. Tighten it and hold it tense. 1 . . . 2 . . . 3. Relax and let go. Good. Breathe in, filling your lungs, and expel your breath slowly. Tighten all the muscles of your hips now, tighter, tighter. 1 . . . 2 . . . 3 . . . Relax and let go. Fine. As you breathe in, notice the relaxation and exhale slowly. Now breathe normally, slowly and deeply. If you feel any tension in any muscle group, you can let it go. Relax and let it go. All the muscles of your body now lie loose, limp and completely relaxed. As you focus on the sound of my voice, your relaxation will progress to an even greater degree. As each muscle relaxes, more relaxation is produced. Your muscles are loose, limp and completely relaxed. Loose, limp, and completely relaxed.

When you were very young, you did not have any breast development. As you grew up and got older you entered a time of body development called puberty. At that time many of your bodily functions where changing so that you would mature and develop into an adult woman. That was when your breasts began their normal growth process.

First, there were changes in the hormone systems in your body. Next, breast tissue and supporting chest muscles developed. Other chemical processes and changes also occurred to help with the development of your breast. For some reason, the process stopped before you developed as much as you would have liked. The reasons why the growth process stopped are no longer important to you. You have learned that your subconscious mind can be used to start the same bodily processes again, the processes necessary for your normal breast development.

Imagine yourself as a young girl. The same physical processes will begin again now exactly as they did when your breasts first started to develop. Your subconscious mind knows exactly when that was, so while you relax deeper and deeper all the bodily processes and changes that are needed to create normal healthy breast growth begin again. Your subconscious mind now will stimulate the same process of breast growth again, just as it did when they first began to develop and this time there is no justifiable reason for the process to stop.

Your breasts now begin to grow and develop until you reach the size you desire. When they reach the size you wish, their growth will stop. During this time of new development you may notice a tingling sensation or a feeling of increased warmth in your breasts. This is normal and is due to the increased blood circulating in the area of your breasts. You want it to happen, you expect it to happen, you feel it happening to you. And now relax deeper and deeper and listen.

It's a beautiful spring day. The smell of spring flowers is in the air. You're twelve years old. What was the world like when you were twelve? What did you look like? What did you think about? What did you feel? Think, feel, remember?

You are standing on the edge of a forest. Squirrels and birds are flitting and scurrying among the trees. The sky is a glorious blue. Big, fluffy, white clouds roll in the sky. On the edge of the forest is a beautiful meadow full of fresh spring flowers and a clear bubbling brook. You run joyously through the meadow, jumping back and forth across the brook. Suddenly, you're at the edge of a large pool of cool fresh water. You're warm and tired from your run through the meadow. You take off your clothes. The sun is hot against your skin. You feel your blood pounding through your body. You take a deep breath and dive into the pool. Your whole body feels tingling and alive from the fresh pure water. You float peacefully on your back and you feel the hot sun on your breasts. You notice that your breasts feel heavier than usual and very, very warm in the sun. You look down at them and you're amazed to see that your breasts have gotten larger than they were before. The skin over your breasts feels tight and pulled as your breasts swell and grow larger. You're feeling excited now. Your heart is beating much faster, in a steady pulsating rhythm. You watch with mounting pleasure as your breasts grow larger and larger with each pounding beat of your heart.

You swim over to some nearby rocks, feeling the water move against your body and you lift yourself up on the warm stone. You feel the warm sun against your wet body. The golden rays of the sun impart a soft glow to your breasts and a soft warm breeze caresses your body with a gentle soothing touch. You rub your naked body all over with a fragrant oil and sense your hands being pushed away from your body as you rub the oil into your growing breasts. You lie down on the rocks and bask nude in the sun, feeling your breasts pulsate larger and larger as the sun's rays become more intense and your breasts grow warmer and warmer. All you can feel is the pressure of your throbbing, growing breasts. You feel young, alive, vibrant, full of health and vigor.

You're home now, back to the present time, and eagerly looking into the mirror to see the incredible change that has occurred in your body. You try on your bra and it just barely covers your breasts. Obviously you'll have to buy a larger bra. You look at your reflection in the mirror and you see your breasts developing and growing right before your eyes. Your whole body is more shapely, better proportioned. It's as though excess fat from other parts of your body has moved into your breasts. Your bra appears to be shrinking, getting smaller and smaller as your breasts grow larger and larger. Your body is developing the beautiful contours you've always wished for. How proud you are that you're a woman, proud of your beautiful body and your large, firm, healthy breasts. You inhale deeply and as your chest fills with air, your breasts swell still larger and larger. Each breath you take enlarges your breasts more and more. You touch your breasts and feel how large they have become. A warm feeling of satisfaction and pleasure grows and multiplies within you. You feel strong, confident, self-assured. Now you look more carefully at your image in the mirror. You see that your breasts are perfectly formed, perfectly healthy, full, round, symmetrical, and firm with a beautiful healthy glow to your skin. You want it to happen, you expect it to happen, you feel it happening to you.

Relax . . . Relax . . . Relax . . . deeper and deeper . . .

Now you imagine yourself at some time in the future after your breasts are their new perfect size. You are getting ready for a party. In the shower you feel your large breasts touch the inside of your upper arms as you move. As you wash your body, you notice how much fuller and heavier your breasts have become. While drying yourself you see that the muscles surrounding your breasts support them beautifully and that the skin of your breasts is soft and smooth and also supports your breasts perfectly. You feel more womanly than you ever have before and your satisfaction and contentment grow stronger and stronger.

You choose a beautiful dress to wear that shows off your breasts in an especially flattering way. You feel comfortable wearing this dress now that your breasts are fully developed and their size and shape please you. At the party, you feel supremely confident about yourself and your body. You're pleased with yourself. Friends and acquaintances compliment you on the wonderful way you look and you sense that they admire your new proportions. You feel confident, proud, and happy, full of vital energy. You now have the body you've always wanted. Your friends want to know what you did to create your new large proportions. You smile and tell them you didn't "do" anything, you simply used the enormous power of your subconscious mind. You imagined yourself with larger breasts and your subconscious mind gave you the body you wished for. No exercise, no surgery, no creams or lotions. Your friends are amazed and continue to compliment you. A great sense of pride and accomplishment comes over you as you realize you have reached your goal. You feel joyful and elated in your new found ability to enlarge your breasts.

At this point you bring yourself back to the present time and you feel you have been transformed. You are completely confident in your ability to maintain the size and development of your breasts.

And now you've come to the end of the session. If you want to return to an alert, clear-headed state, do so as you count to three. On the other hand, if you would like to go to sleep, do so. Don't count to three and just drift off to sleep. Whether you open your eyes now or later, you will feel better for having enjoyed this deep relaxation. It has renewed and refreshed you. Now if you're returning to an alert clear-headed state, count to three, wake up your body, and open your eyes. 1 . . . 2 . . . 3.

If you would like to go to sleep, relax deeply, deeper than before. As your relaxation becomes deeper and deeper, of course, you will become sleepier and sleepier. Perhaps you will be asleep in just a few moments — sleep peacefully, restfully, and be renewed and refreshed while you sleep. When you awaken, be pleased and happy with yourself, because even while you sleep, your breasts are enlarging, becoming fuller and firmer. Now sleep . . . sleep . . . sleep.

What Happens Next?

You have completed your first full conditioning session to enlarge your breasts. You have used the power of your mind to set in motion the creative forces that will bring about exactly what you have visualized. What happens now? Do you rush off to measure? Try another session? Read another chapter?

The answer is you live life just as you always have, do just what you normally feel like doing. Nothing has happened to warrant special attention or change of routine. Watching yourself now will prove nothing, because the transformation that has started in you has started in your subconscious. You cannot be conscious about the subconscious.

Natural Breast Enlargement

Chart and Measuring Instructions

When using the Natural Breast Enlargement method you may find it helpful to keep a daily record of the number of times you use the program. The best way to realize your progress is to see it on your chart. You can make up one of your own or use the one I have provided.

Begin by entering the date you start using Natural Breast Enlargement techniques. From this day on your breast enlargement will begin officially. Place a small check in the column "Number of times recording was played" for each day you use Natural Breast Enlargement suggestions. If you prefer, enter the time of day that you use the program.

You will be able to tell that your breasts are enlarging by the way they look and feel. You may also want to keep a weekly record of your development. You can do this best by taking the correct breast measurements using the following procedures.

1. Take your measurements at the same time of day since your body weight fluctuates during any twenty-four hour period, depending on your own metabolic cycles.

2. Be sure to measure after a normal exhalation. (You don't want a deep breath causing a false increase!)

3. Stand up straight when you measure, since your posture may affect your proportions. If you wish, have someone help you take the measurements. Then you don't have to have "eyes in the back of your head" to see if the tape is straight and level.

4. Record the following measurements:

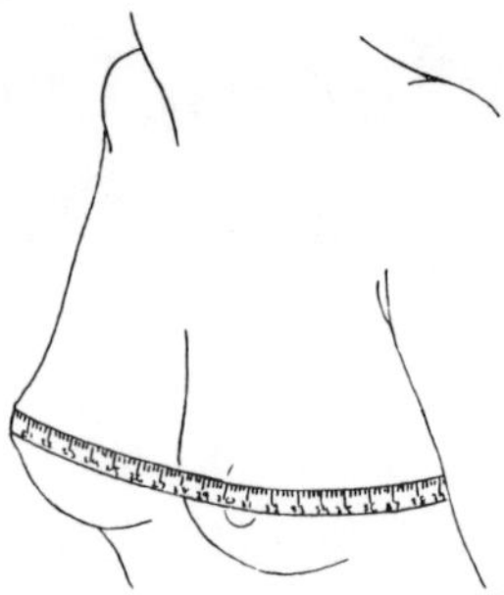

(A). BREAST MEASUREMENT

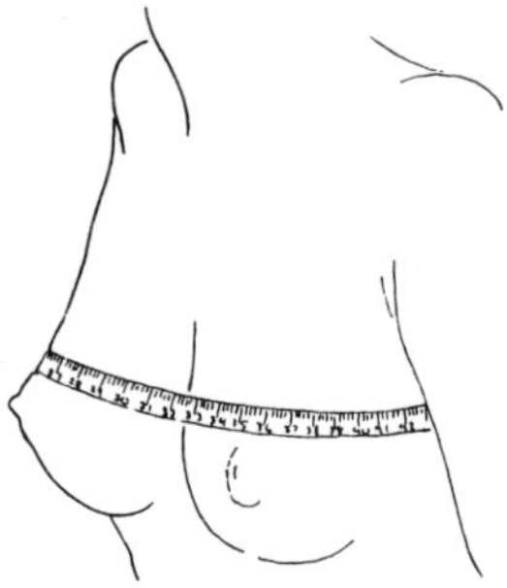

(C). UPPER BREAST MEASUREMENT

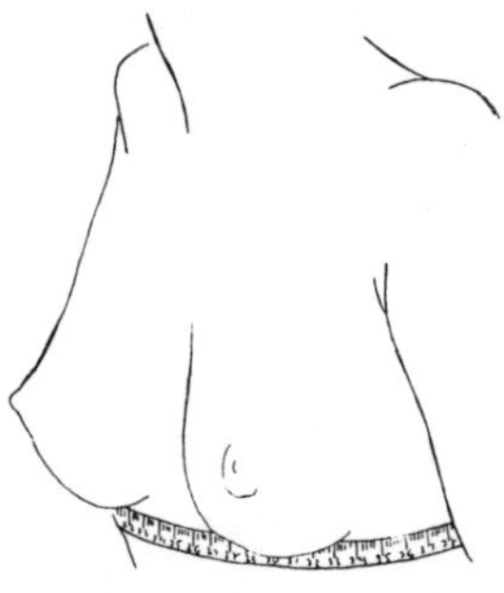

(B). CHEST MEASUREMENT

A. Measure around your chest and breasts at their fullest point at the nipple line. Be careful not to pull too tightly. It's best to measure with the nipple flat against your breast.

B. Measure around your chest right below the base of the cup of your breast.

C. Measure around your chest, above your breasts where they begin to swell away from your chest. For a woman of average size, this measurement is approximately two inches above the nipple. For a large-breasted woman the tape will be further than two inches from the nipple; for a small-breasted woman the tape will be closer than two inches from the nipple.

D. Record your weight at the same time you are measuring your breasts. A gain or loss of five pounds is acceptable during the course of the program and will not affect your results.
E. (Optional.) Measure around your waist. Many women have reported a shaping effect throughout their bodies while using these techniques. You may become smaller in your waist.
F. (Optional.) Measure your hips for the same reason.

5. Record your measurements and your weight once a week for twelve to sixteen weeks.

If you wish, once you have reached your desired result you can maintain your increase by periodically listening to or reading your suggestions. However, I have not found that any reinforcement was needed for maintaining breast increase.

Progress Chart

Starting Date: ____________________

Week	Number of times recording was played Days 1	2	3	4	5	6	7	Measurements in inches A	B	C	D	E	F
1													
2													
3													
4													
5													
6													
7													
8													
9													
10													
11													
12													
13													
14													
15													
16													

Measurements

	Before Starting Program	Completion of Program	Net Change
A — Breast	______	______	______
B — Chest	______	______	______
C — Upper Breast	______	______	______
D — Weight (Optional)	______	______	______
E — Waist	______	______	______
F — Hips	______	______	______

REFERENCES

Arnold, M. D. On the mechanism of suggestion and hypnosis. *Journal of Abnormal and Social Psychology,* 1946, *41,* 107 - 128.

Ayalah, D. & Weinstock, I. J. *Breasts – women speak about their breasts and their lives.* New York, Summit Books, 1979.

Baker, J. L.; Kolin, I.; & Bartlett, E.S. Psychosexual dynamics of patients undergoing mammary augmentation. *Plastic and Reconstructive Surgery – Psychosexual Dynamics,* 1974, *53* (6), 652 - 659.

Barber, T. X. Hypnosis, suggestion and psychosomatic phenomena: a new look from the standpoint of recent experimental studies. In J. L. Fosshage and P. Alson, (Eds.), *Healing: Implications for Psychotherapy.* New York: Behavioral Publications, in press.

Barber, T. X. Introduction to self-control: temperature, biofeedback, hypnosis, yoga and relaxation. *Biofeedback and self-control.* 1975/76, Chicago: Aldine Publishing Co., 1976, xiii - xxix.

Barber, T. X. Physiological effects of "hypnotic suggestions": A critical review of recent research (1960 - 1964). *Psychological Bulletin,* 1965, *63* (4), 201 - 219.

Barber, T. X. Responding to "hypnotic" suggestions: an introspective report. *The American Journal of Clinical Hypnosis.* 1975, *18,* 6 - 22.

Barber, T. X. & DeMoor, W. A theory of hypnotic induction procedures. *The American Journal of Clinical Hypnosis,* 1972, *15* (2), 112 - 135.

Barber, D. E.; et al., "Bleeding" of silicone from bag-gel breast implants, and its clinical relation to fibrous capsule reaction. *Plastic and Reconstructive Surgery.* 1978, *61,* 836 - 841.

Bem, S. Verbal self-control: the establishment of effective self-instruction. *Journal of Experimental Pyschology.* 1967, *74,* 485 - 491.

Benson, H. *The relaxation response.* New York: William Morrow and Company, Inc., 1975.

Berscheid, E.; Walster, E.; & Bohrnstedt, G. Body-image: A psychology today questionnaire. *Psychology Today,* July, 1972, 58 - 64.

Berscheid, E.; Walster, E.; & Bohrnstedt, G. The happy American body: A survey report. *Psychology Today,* November, 1973, 119 - 131.

Blakeslee, T. R. Your unconscious, dreamy brain: it's all RIGHT, research finds. *Science Digest,* 1980, *1,* 30 - 33.

Brazel, J. A. & Blizzard, R. M. The influence of the endocrine glands upon growth and development. In R. H. Williams (Ed.), *Textbook of Endocrinology* (5th ed.), Philadelphia: W. B. Saunders, 1974.

Brown, B. B. *New mind, new body.* New York: Harper and Row, Publishers, 1974.

Bry, A. *Directing the movies of your mind.* New York: Harper and Row Publishers, Inc., 1978.

Budzynski, T. H. Some applications of biofeedback produced twilight states. *Biofeedback and Self-Control 1972.* 1973, 145 - 151.

Capozzi, A.; et al. Distant migration of silicone gel from a ruptured breast implant. *Plastic and Reconstructive Surgery.* 1978, *62,* 302 - 303.

Cheek, D. B. & LeCron, L. M. *Clinical hypnotherapy.* New York: Grune and Stralton, 1968.

Coe, E. C.; Allen, J. L.; Krug, W. M.; & Worzmann, A. G. Goal-directed fantasy in hypnotic responsiveness: Skill, item, wording or both? *The International Journal of Clinical and Experimental Hypnosis,* 1974, *22* (2), 157 - 166.

Damaser, E. C.; Shor, R. E.; & Orne, M. T. Physiological effects during hypnotically requested emotions. *Psychosomatic Medicine,* 1963, *25* (4), 334 - 343.

Desaxe, B. M. Breast augmentation: Results in a series of 150 cases. *South African Medical Journal,* 1974, *48,* 737 - 740.

Deutsch, F. Der gusunde und der kranke korper, in psychoanalylicher bertrachtung. Cited by H. F. Dunbar, *Emotions and Bodily Changes,* (4th ed.) New York: Columbia University Press, 1954.

DiCara, L. V. Learning in the autonomic nervous system. *Scientific American,* 1970, *222,* 30 - 39.

Druss, R. Changes in body image following augmentation breast surgery. *International Journal of Psychoanalytic Psychotherapy.* 1973, *2* (2), 248 - 256.

Edelman, R. J. Effects of progressive relaxation on autonomic processes. *Journal of Clinical Psychology,* 1970, *26,* 421 - 425.

Edgerton, M. T. & McClary, A. R. Augmentation mammoplasty. *Plastic and Reconstructive Surgery,* 1958, *21* (4), 279 - 305.

Edwards, B. *Drawing on the right side of the brain.* New York, J. P. Tarcher, Inc., 1979.

Eisenberg, H. V. Rupture of a silicone bag-gel breast implant by closed compression capsulotomy. *Plastic and Reconstructive Surgery.* 1977, *59,* 849 - 850.

Erickson, M. H. Breast development possibly influenced by hypnosis: Two instances and the therapeutic results. *American Journal of Clinical Hypnosis.* 1960, *3,* 157 - 159.

Erickson, M. H. Pseudo-orientation in the time as an hypnotherapeutic procedure. *Journal of Clinical and Experimental Hypnosis,* 1954, *2,* 261 - 283.

Erickson, M. H.; Rossi, E. L.; & Rossi, S. *Hypnotic realities.* New York: Irvington Publishers, 1976.

Evans, F. J. Suggestibility in the normal waking state. *Psychology Bulletin,* 1967, *67,* 114.

Fisher, S. *Body consciousness: you are what you feel.* Englewood, N.J.: Prentice-Hall, 1973.

Fisher, S. Aniseikonic perception by women of their own breasts. *Perceptual and Motor Skill,* 1973, *36,* 1021 - 1022.

Ford, L. F. & Yeager, C. L. Changes in the electroencephalogram in subjects under hypnosis. *Disorders of the Nervous System,* 1948, *9,* 190 - 194.

Gadpaille, W. J. *The cycles of sex.* New York: Scribner and Sons, 1975.

Gottschalk, L. A. Self-induced visual imagery, affect arousal, and autonomic correlates. *Psychosomatics,* 1974, *4,* 166.

Graham, C. & Leibowitz, H. W. The effect of suggestion on visual acuity. *International Journal of Clinical and Experimental Hypnosis,* 1972, *20,* 169 - 186.

Graham, D. T.; Kabler, J. D.; & Graham, F. D. Physiological response to the suggestion of attitudes specific for hives and hypertension. *Psychosomatic Medicine,* 1962, *24,* 159 - 169.

Graham, D. T.; Stern, J. A.; & Winokur, G. Experimental investigation of the specificity of attitude hypnosis in psychosomatic disease. *Psychosomatic Medicine,* 1958.

Gray, H. *Gray's anatomy.* New York: Bounty Books, 1977.

Green, E. & Green, A. Mind training, ESP, hypnosis and voluntary control of internal states. *The Academy of Parapsychology and Medicine,* 1973.

Green, E. E.; Green, A. M.; & Walters, E. D. Self-regulation of internal states. *Progress of cybernetics: Proceedings of the International Congress of Cybernetics.* London: Gordon and Breach, 1970, 1299 - 1317.

Green, E.; Green, A.; & Walters, E. Voluntary control of internal states: psychological and physiological. *Journal of Transpersonal Psychology,* 190, *2* (1), 1 - 16.

Groddeck, G. Ueber die psychoanalyse des organischen im menschen. Cited by H. F. Dunbar, *Emotions and Bodily Changes,* (4th ed.). New York: Columbia University Press, 1954.

Gruber, R. P.; et al. The pressures generated by closed capsulotomies of augmented breasts. *Plastic and Reconstructive Surgery,* 1978, *62,* 379 - 380.

Hadfield, J. A. The influence of suggestions on body temperature. *Lancet,* 1920, *2,* 68 - 69.

Hammer, M. The directed daydream technique. *Psychotherapy: Theory, Research and Practice,* 1967, *4,* 173 - 181.

Hartland, J. The general principles of suggestion. *The American Journal of Clinical Hypnosis,* 1967, 9 (3), 211 - 219.

Harwood, L. R. Changes in visual acuity in myopic subjects during hypnosis. Paper presented at the annual meeting of the American Academy of Optometry, Miami, December 13, 1970.

Hayes, H. Breast implants and possible late hematogenous infection. *Plastic and Reconstructive Surgery,* 1977, *60,* 104.

Hilgard, J. P. *Personality and hypnosis.* Chicago: University of Chicago Press, 1970.

Hirose, S.; Hirayama, D.; & Ikemi, Y. The influence of emotional stress on the blood liver flow. *Kyushu Journal of Medical Science,* 1961, *12,* 319 - 323.

Hitschmann, E. Psychoanalyse trotz hormonen. Cited by H. F. Dunbar, *Emotions and Bodily Changes,* (4th ed.), New York: Columbia University Press, 1954.

Hutton, F. A. Augmentation mammoplasty. Fibrous capsular contracture and other complications. *Journal of the Kansas Medical Society,* 1978, *79,* 205 - 206.

Ikemi, Y.; and Nakagawa, S. A psychosomatic study of contagious dermatitus. *Kyshu Journal of Medical Science,* 1962, *13,* 335 - 350.

Johnson, R. F. Q. & Barber, T. X. Hypnosis, suggestions, and warts: an experimental investigation implicating the importance of "believed-in" efficacy. Mass: Medfield Foundation, 1977.

Kelley, C. R. Psychological factors in myopia, Doctoral dissertation, New School for Social Research, 1958.

Kelly, G. F. Guided fantasy as a counseling technique with youth. *Journal of Counseling Psychology.* 1972, *19* (5), 355 - 361.

Klemperer, E. Changes of the body image in hypnoanalysis. *Journal of Clinical and Experimental Hypnosis,* 1945, *2,* 157 - 162.

Kolin, I. S.; Baker, J. L. & Bartlett, E. S. Sex after breast augmentation. *Medical Aspects of Human Sexuality,* 1967, *10,* 123.

Kroger, W. S. *Clinical and experimental hypnosis.* Philadelphia: J. B. Lippincott, 1963.

Kroger, W. S. & Fezler, W. D. *Hypnosis and behavior modification: imagery conditioning.* Philadelphia: J. B. Lippincott, 1976.

Lang, P. Autonomic control of learning to play the internal organs. *Psychology Today,* October, 1970, 37 - 41.

LeCron, L. M. A study of age regression under hypnosis. In L. M. LeCron (ed.), *Experimental hypnosis.* New York: Citadel Press, 1965.

LeCron, L. M. Breast development through hypnotic suggestion. *Journal of the American Society of Psychosomatic Dentistry and Medicine,* 1969, *16,* 58 - 61.

Levitsky, A. The constructive realistic fantasy. *The American Journal of Hypnosis: Clinical, Experimental, Theoretical,* 1966, 9 (1), 52 - 55.

Lloyd, C. W. Problems associated with sexual maturation and lactation. In C. W. Lloyd (ed.), *Human reproduction and sexual behavior.* Philadelphia: Lea and Febiger, 1964.

Lloyd, C. W. & Leathem, J. H. Growth and development of the breast and lactation. In C. W. Lloyd (ed.), *Human reproduction and sexual behavior.* Philadelphia: Lea & Febiger, 1964.

Maltz, M. *Psychocybernetics.* New York: Simon & Schuster, 1960.

Martin, I. & Grosz, H. J. Hypnotically induced emotions: Autonomic and skeletal muscle activity in patients with affective illnesses. *Archives of General Psychiatry,* 1964, *11,* 203 - 213.

Menninger, K. A. Somatic correlations with the unconscious repudiation of feminity in women. *Journal of Nervous and Mental Disease,* 1939, *89,* 514 - 527.

Miller, E. E. *Selective awareness.* 1975.

Miller, N. E. Learning of glandular and visceral responses. *Current Status of Physiological Psychology,* 1972.

Miller, N. E. Learning of visceral and glandular responses. *Science,* 1969, *163,* 434 - 445.

Mohr, F. Psychophysisch behandlungsmethoden. Cited by H. F. Dunbar, *Emotions and bodily changes* (4th ed.). New York: Columbia University Press, 1954.

Murphy, J. *The power of your subconscious mind.* Englewood Cliffs, N.J.: Prentice-Hall, Inc., 1963.

Mutke, P. H. C. *Selective awareness.* Millbrae, CA: Celestial Arts, 1977.

Mutke, P. H. C. Self-image and breast development. *Selective awareness.* Millbrae, CA: Celestial Arts, 1977, 149 - 156.

Mutke, P. H. C. Research paper on the subject of mental techniques for breast development, presented to the Department of Neuropsychiatry, University of California, Los Angeles, February 28, 1971.

Mysior, A. Shifting from conceptual to visual problem solving facilitated by hypnosis. *The American Journal of Clinical Hypnosis,* 1971, *14* (2), 97 - 101.

Nașher, M. & White, M. Beauty and the breast: a 60% complication rate for an operation you don't need. *MS,* September 1977, pp 53 - 54, 84 - 88.

Ohlsen, L., et al. Augmentation mammoplasty: A surgical and psychiatric evaluation of the results. *Annals of Plastic Surgery,* 1979, *2,* 42 - 52.

Ornstein, R. E. *The psychology of consciousness.* San Francisco: W. H. Freeman & Co., 1972.

Oyle, I. *The healing mind.* Celestial Arts: Millbrae, CA, 1975.

Packard, J. Breast enlargement with three types of hypnotic suggestions. California State University, at Sacramento, 1979.

Paul, G. L. Physiological effects of relaxation training and hypnotic suggestion. *Journal of Abnormal Psychology.* 1969, *74,* 425.

Reichlen, S. Neuroendocrinology. In R. H. Williams (ed.), *Textbook of endocrinology,* (4th ed.). Philadelphia: W. B. Saunders, 1968.

Renneker, R.; et al. Psychoanalytic exploration of the breast. *Psychosomatic Medicine,* 1963, *25,* 106 - 123.

Richardson, A. *Mental imagery.* New York: Springer Publishing Co., 1969.

Rosenthal, S. *Cosmetic surgery: a consumer's guide.* Philadelphia: J. B. Lippincott Co., 1976.

Schneider, A. M. & Tarshis, B. *Physiological psychology.* New York: Random House, 1975.

Schwartz, G. E. Biofeedback, self-regulation, and the patterning of physiological processes. *American Scientist,* 1975, *63,* 314 - 324.

Sheehan, P. W. *The function and nature of imagery.* New York: Academic Press, 1972.

Shipley, R. H.; O'Donnell, J. M.; & Bader, K. F. Personality characteristics of women seeking breast augmentation. *Plastic and Reconstructive Surgery,* 1977, *60* (3), 369 - 376.

Simonton, O. C.; Mathews-Simonton, S.; & Creighton, J. *Getting well again.* Los Angeles: J. P. Tarcher, Inc. 1978.

Smith, A. *Powers of mind.* New York: Random House, Inc. 1975.

Snyder, G. B. Complications of augmentation mammoplasty. In W. C. Grabb and J. W. Smith (eds.), *Plastic surgery.* Boston: Little, Brown and Company, 1968, 834 - 844.

Spanos, N. P. & Barber, T. X. Cognitive activity during "hypnotic suggestibility": goal-directed fantasy and the experience of nonvolition. *Journal of Personality,* in press.

Spanos, N. Goal-directed fantasy and the performance of hypnotic test suggestions. *Psychiatry,* 1971, *34,* 86 - 96.

Spanos, N. P. & Barber, T. X. Toward a convergence in hypnosis research, *American Psychologist,* 1974, *29* (7), 500 - 511.

Staib, A. R. & Logan, D. R. Hypnotic stimulation of breast growth. *American Journal of Clinical Hypnosis,* 1977, *19* (4), 201 - 208.

Stallings, J. O. A new you: *How plastic surgery can change your life.* New York: Mason/Charter, 1977.

Stern, J. A.; Winoker, G.; Graham, D. T.; & Graham, F. K. Alteration in physiological measure during experimentally induced attitudes. *Journal of Psychosomatic Research.* 1961, *5,* 73 - 82.

Tarlau, M. & Smalheiser, I. Personality patterns in patients with malignant tumors of the breast and cervix. *Psychosomatic Medicine,* 1951, *13,* 117 - 121.

Willard, R. D. Breast enlargement through visual imagery and hypnosis. *American Journal of Clinical Hypnosis,* 1977, *19* (4), 195 - 200.

Williams, J. W. Stimulation of breast growth by hypnosis. *The Journal of Sex Research,* 1974, *10* (4), 316 - 326.

Wilson, D. L. *Natural bust enlargement with total mind power. How to use the other 90° of your mind to increase the size of your breasts.* Calif: Total Mind Power Institute, 1979.

Wilson, D. L. *Total beauty through total mind power – how to use the other 90° of your mind to improve your beauty.* In process of publication, 1979.

Wilson, D. L. *Total mind power – how to use the other 90° of your mind.* New York: Berkley Publishing Corp., 1978.

Acknowledgements

I wish to offer sincere thanks and deep appreciation to the following individuals from whom I have received personal and professional support and guidance. They all have contributed to the present effort.

Dr. Beata Jencks of the Department of Psychology at the University of Utah, who taught me the value of autogenic training and added her support and encouragement to my maiden efforts in using hypnosis.

Dr. James Alexander of the same department of psychology, who took a chance on an untried undergraduate and piloted me through my experiences at the Women's Facility of the Utah State Prison.

The thirty-one women who took thirteen weeks out of their busy schedules and committed themselves to completing the study. Without them there would be no book!

Dr. Helene Burgess of the Department of Psychology at California State University, Sacramento, whose research expertise and editing skill transformed the rough drafts of my master's thesis into recognizable form.

Dr. Neal Grossen, also of the Department of Psychology, CSUS, who assisted me in unraveling the intricacies of the statistical data and guided me in their proper interpretation.

Carl Thompson, special friend and colleague, who continuously provides unflagging support and who generously furnished the professional setting in which my research was conducted.

Dr. Alvyn Freed and his wife Marge, who created the opportunity for me to share what I learned. Without their steady encouragement and enthusiasm this book would never have been attempted.

Suzanne Mikesell, my editor, who managed to significantly reduce the gap between my thinking and my writing and thereby maintain the internal consistency of the manuscript.

Marna Miller, Dee Kiene, Barbara Anderson, and Carolyn Kiene who typed, proofread, and then typed some more, always under pressure to meet various deadlines.

Richard Kiene, the artist, whose patient willingness to redraw as concepts changed form was greatly appreciated.

Finally to dear friends and loved ones, particularly my children, for their sacrifices, patient support, understanding and encouragement, not only during the preparation of the manuscript, but throughout the past few years of my life.

JOAN PACKARD is a licensed marriage and family counselor with Life Awareness Associates in Sacramento, California. She received her Master's Degree in Psychology from California State University, where she conducted an extensive research project on breast augmentation through deep relaxation techniques involving 32 subjects. She is a member of the California Psychological Association, the American Institute of Hypnosis and is President-elect of the Sacramento Academy of Professional and Clinical Hypnosis.

Natural Breast Enlargement, her first book, is a straightforward, tasteful, and non-threatening presentation based on scientifically valid research using professional techniques. Written for women of all ages, *Natural Breast Enlargement* shows how using a person's dreams to tap an inner source of power can affect a change, not only in breast size, but in lifelong goals as well.

WILLIAM S. KROGER, M.D. is a respected authority on the use of suggestion and hypnosis in medical therapy. He has taught the basic principles of hypnosis for forty years to more than 100,000 physicians throughout the world. His books, *Clinical and Experimental Hypnosis* and *Hypnosis and Behavior Modification,* have become standard reference works in the field of psychosomatic medicine and hypnotherapy.

Dr. Kroger is a Clinical Professor, Department of Anesthesiology, University of California Los Angeles School of Medicine; Consultant to the Pain Clinic, U.C.L.A.; and a Consulting Psychiatrist at City of Hope Medical Center, Century City and Los Angeles New Hospitals, California. He founded the Institute for Comprehensive Medicine in Beverly Hills, California.